Remaking Health Care
in America

Stephen M. Shortell
Robin R. Gillies
David A. Anderson
Karen Morgan Erickson
John B. Mitchell

Remaking Health Care in America

Building Organized
Delivery Systems

Jossey-Bass Publishers
San Francisco

Substantial discounts on bulk quantities of Jossey-Bass books are available to corporations, professional associations, and other organizations. For details and discount information, contact the special sales department at Jossey-Bass Inc., Publishers (415) 433–1740; Fax (800) 605–2665.

For sales outside the United States, please contact your local Simon & Schuster International Office.

Jossey-Bass Web address: http://www.josseybass.com

 Manufactured in the United States of America on Lyons Falls Pathfinder Tradebook. This paper is acid-free and 100 percent totally chlorine-free.

Library of Congress Cataloging-in-Publication Data

Remaking health care in America: building organized delivery systems/
 [Stephen M. Shortell . . . et al.]
  p. cm.—(The Jossey-Bass health series)
  Includes bibliographical references and index.
  ISBN 0-7879-0227-6 (alk. paper)
   1. Medical care—United States. 2. Health facilities—United States—Affiliations.
 3. Health services administration—United States. I. Shortell, Stephen M.
 (Stephen Michael), date. II. Series.
 RA395.A3R46 1996
 362.1'0973—dc20   95-46557
                                                                        CIP

HB Printing   10 9 8 7 6 5 4 3   FIRST EDITION

Contents

Preface

In 1990 we published *Strategic Choices for America's Hospitals: Managing Change in Turbulent Times*. Based on systematic study of eight multihospital systems over three years, we concluded that these largely successful systems had added relatively little overall value on almost any dimension of performance. The primary reasons were twofold. First, these systems were still relatively loose collections of hospitals that lacked the properties of "systemness," whereby competencies and capabilities are shared throughout the system and efforts are made to reduce unnecessary duplication and fragmentation. Second, these systems were primarily concerned with creating administrative economies of scope and scale and were not yet ready to take on the difficult task of restructuring patient care activities across the continuum of care, a process we call *clinical integration*.

Recognizing that multihospital systems as they were structured at the time would not be able to address the looming changes in payment and health care reform initiatives, I became interested in conducting a follow-up study of how these or similar systems were attempting to adjust to the new realities of both the marketplace and health reform. At approximately the same time, I was visited in the spring of 1990 by Jack Newman and Bob Schimmel of KPMG Peat Marwick. They expressed interest in conducting a study of the new generation of health systems. At a subsequent session we met with Dave Anderson, the firm's designated "closet academic" selected to head up the KPMG team. We agreed on the general content of the study, the approach, and the types of systems we wanted to examine.

The study was initially viewed with skepticism and even cynicism in some quarters. People questioned whether the cultures, goals, motivations, and objectives of a consulting firm, eleven different provider systems, and a university were sufficiently compatible to execute the study. Were the provider systems far enough along in their integration efforts and "mature enough" to be studied? Did KPMG really understand the difference between research and consulting? Could the university-based investigators remain independent and objective in their analysis given that the study was funded by the provider systems themselves? How would the academicians reconcile their need for additional analysis and verification with the providers' demand for timely feedback? Was there sufficient overlap in the study teams and participants' cultures and values for a meaningful study to endure over the planned three years?

The answer to all of the questions was a resounding yes, which we believe is attributable to four factors. First, the fact that each health system supported the study in the amount of $50,000 per year provided the right financial incentives for all parties. The study systems were motivated to cooperate, providing ready access to data and information and agreeing to two summers of on-site interviews; the study team felt obligated to produce analysis and results in a timely fashion to satisfy their paying customers.

A second major reason for the study's success was the commitment, foresight, and leadership of the system CEOs and strategic planners—the latter of whom served as the study's research advisory group. The CEOs understood both the educational value of the study itself and how the study results could be used to advance strategic initiatives throughout their systems. They committed their organizations to full involvement. The research advisory group

members were invaluable guides for the study team: they helped pri-
oritize issues and develop measures, and they suggested strategies
for collecting, presenting, and disseminating data.

A third reason for the success of the study was the chemistry
achieved among the KPMG and Northwestern study team members. We believed we were working at the cutting edge of the newly
emerging health care system in the United States and had the rare
opportunity to distill major lessons from the systematic study of
eleven different systems operating in eleven different markets
throughout the country. A sense of adventure, excitement, and
"mission" permeated the team as we met regularly over the course
of the four years to develop working hypotheses, design data collection instruments, plan meetings with participants, discuss the
analysis and implications of our findings, and, finally, plan and write
this book. We appreciated each other's skills and insights, and at
times it was difficult to distinguish who among us were the "acade-
mics" and who were the "consultants."

The final factor contributing to the study's success was the accelerated growth of managed care, capitated payment, and various
health care reform initiatives at both the state and national levels.
These environmental forces intensified each study system's efforts
to develop a more cost-effective, integrated continuum of care that
could meet the demands of purchasers. As a result, the study took
on an almost day-to-day relevance as findings and recommendations
emerged.

None of the above should suggest to the reader that the study
was easy to do or that there were not disagreements, frustrations,
and disappointments. There were several instances in which the
study systems would have liked to have had results sooner than we
were able to produce them. Some of the early feedback reports were
not "user friendly." The study team was not always able to respond
to special requests for discussion or presentation of findings. There
were also honest disagreements about how much and what kinds of
data should be collected—particularly in constructing the objective

measures of physician-system and clinical integration. Nonetheless, the financial incentives of the study, the importance of the issues addressed, and the quality of the people involved enabled us to work through these challenges in a satisfactory and, in some cases, exemplary fashion.

Purpose of the Book

This is a time of great skepticism and unrest in the health care world. Conflicting financial incentives, escalating cost-containment pressures, often unrealistic patient expectations, and the lack of a coherent national health care policy are beginning to grind down providers, insurers, employers, and consumers alike. As a result, such micro-managerial innovations as continuous quality improvement/ total quality management (CQI/TQM) and macro-organizational innovations such as integrated or organized delivery systems are viewed with suspicion. Are they just another passing fad? Do they have any substance? What do we really know about them? What impact are they having? These are all relevant questions. But we believe they should be answered through systematic study of what works and doesn't work under varying circumstances. Knowledge-building is important to community-building. It is in this spirit that the Health System Integration Study and this book were undertaken.

It is important to position the study and the book within the historical evolution of the U.S. health care system. From the delivery or provider perspective, four stages might be noted. The first stage was marked by the proliferation of individual hospitals and physicians stimulated by the post–World War II Hill-Burton program to fund hospital construction and by the growth of medical schools and medical education. Health care was often referred to as a "cottage industry," comprising thousands of small physician practices and local community hospitals. The second stage began in the late 1960s and early 1970s with the emergence of both investor-owned and not-for-profit multihospital systems. The primary focus of these systems was on achieving economies of scale, developing a stronger capital base, and solidifying market share, particularly across wider geographic areas. In the late 1980s and into the present, a third stage has emerged in which the multihospital systems and other groups are attempting to become integrated or *organized delivery systems*, concentrating on primarily local or regional markets. There are also increasing linkages with insurance companies and managed care organizations. As managed care pressures grow, multihospital systems have seen the need to organize and manage the entire continuum from primary care to hospice care differently in order to effectively serve enrolled populations. Further, as health care delivery continues to move away from the hospital as organizational center, a number of integrated delivery systems are organized around physician groups or large multispecialty clinics.

We believe that the seeds of a fourth stage are beginning to emerge that will transform the current integrated or organized delivery systems into what we call *community health care management systems*. In this fourth stage, the delivery of personal health care services represented by the organized delivery system will begin to focus on community-wide health care needs through alliances, coalitions, linkages, and partnerships with public health and community and social service agencies. Although this book is primarily about organized delivery systems in the third stage of evolution, we attempt to anticipate the fourth stage by suggesting some of the components needed for achieving an effective community health care management system. The third stage, characterized by the organized delivery system, brings together *medicine and management* in ways seldom seen before. In the fourth stage, medicine, management, and *public health* will be brought together as they never have been before. Moving from stage three to stage four will be an enormous challenge because it involves moving from a personal health care system that is not very well integrated to a community health system that is, in some respects, virtually nonexistent!

Organized delivery systems must be seen as an intermediate form preceding the development of the community health care management system. The challenges are to (1) overcome the extreme fragmentation that characterizes the present delivery of health care services, (2) learn how to build community, (3) develop the competencies and capabilities required for a community health care management system, and (4) establish a local and national health policy that supports the transformation efforts. These four challenges are discussed as recurring themes throughout this book.

Readers will note that we prefer the term *organized delivery system* to the more frequently used *integrated delivery system* because we believe integration is an end state that few, if any, current systems have achieved. The term has been used too loosely in the professional literature and media to describe combinations of hospital, physician, and insurer arrangements that may exist on paper but are, in fact, anything but integrated. Hospitals, physicians, insurers, and other entities are, however, trying to *organize* themselves to achieve a greater degree of coordinated care across the continuum; hence, we feel that our term more accurately describes the study systems.

Overview of the Contents

The goal of developing a community health care management system is a major theme of *Remaking Health Care in America*, and the book systematically identifies the basic building blocks of such a system, including population-based planning; functional, physician-system, and clinical integration; and a continuous cycle of total quality management to continuously improve health care services for populations. In addition, the book discusses the broader-based public policy issues that can provide incentives or disincentives for creating a community health care management system. The book links theory with action in developing a practical approach to implementing a new paradigm of health care delivery.

Chapter One centers on the theme of fragmentation and discusses the need for a more holistic, integrated approach to the delivery of health care in the United States.

Chapter Two presents two scenarios to illustrate what an ideal health care system would look like, and introduces the concept of a holographic organization—one in which the whole is embedded into each of the parts.

Chapter Three presents the overall conceptual framework for the study. This framework suggests that an organization's vision, values, leadership, and strategies help to promote the integration of functions, which in turn promotes the integration of physicians with systems, which is in turn critical to achieving clinical integration. Chapter Three also introduces the eleven systems studied and briefly highlights the study's approach. (Further details are provided in Resources A and B.)

Chapter Four examines the extent to which each system integrates its finances, human resources, strategic planning, information systems, total quality management, and related functions. Particular attention is given to the importance of information systems and total quality management.

Chapter Five looks at the extent to which physicians are integrated into systems of care. It emphasizes the importance of physician leadership development programs and of taking flexible, pluralistic approaches to working with physicians. Practical cases illustrate successful strategies for involving physicians.

Chapter Six examines clinical integration—the extent to which patient care services are coordinated across people, facilities, functions, activities, and time. Particular attention is given to planning for clinical integration, holding people accountable, and the role of total quality management and information systems in promoting clinical integration. Again, several case studies are presented to illustrate the major points.

Chapter Seven describes what is needed to manage and govern the organized delivery system. It discusses the challenge of overcoming the reliance on the hospital as the center of health care delivery and examines the need to create cross-boundary, cross-functional management and governance roles. The chapter also emphasizes issues related to control. Again, case studies illustrate the major points.

Chapter Eight highlights the public policy issues related to encouraging more organized delivery systems and holding such systems accountable. The topics of antitrust, personnel licensure, financial incentives, and related issues are raised. The chapter also discusses special issues related to academic medical centers, vulnerable populations, and the delivery of health care in rural America.

Audiences for the Book

There are four major audiences for the book: health services executives and clinical leaders; insurers and payers; health care policy makers at the state and federal levels; and health services researchers. For health services executives and clinical leaders, the book provides practical suggestions and examples for developing more cost-effective organized delivery systems. Chapters Four through Seven, dealing with issues of functional, physician-system, and clinical integration as well as management and governance, will be of particular interest. For insurers and payers, the book's many examples, recommendations, best practices, and key success factors provide important criteria for contracting and developing payer-provider alliances. Chapter Five, on physician-system integration, and Chapter Six, on clinical integration, will be of particular interest to purchasers. For policy makers, Chapter Eight is "must reading," as it highlights various options for encouraging the development of organized systems and addresses important accountability issues. For our health services research colleagues, the book represents the first systematic empirical assessment of the movement toward more integrated systems and, as such, provides a conceptual and empirical base for further work. Resource B summarizes the study's extensive data collection tools and methodologies. We hope that all readers will at least skim Chapters One and Two, which highlight the fundamental problems of our current health system and develop the concept of the community health care management system.

Creating organized delivery systems that can be used as a foundation for developing community health care management systems is a difficult task. One must recognize that all of the systems studied are in the relatively early stages of integration, particularly in regard to clinical integration. Much experimentation and learning needs to occur. Further, although the issues and challenges are raised within the context of the U.S. health care system, we believe that the same underlying dynamics and forces are at work in many health care systems throughout the world, particularly those of Australia, Canada, Germany, Great Britain, and New Zealand. There is much that the United States can learn from these other countries and, it is hoped, much that they can learn from our early efforts to fundamentally transform the way in which we organize and deliver health services.

March 1996

Stephen M. Shortell
Evanston, Illinois

Robin R. Gillies
Evanston, Illinois

David A. Anderson
Chicago, Illinois

Karen Morgan Erickson
Minneapolis, Minnesota

John B. Mitchell
Minneapolis, Minnesota

Acknowledgments

• •

This study could not have happened without the extraordinary support and cooperation from the participating systems. This includes corporate board members, executives, and staff, and members affiliated with the systems' many operating units. Their willingness to share data, information, and their own insights gave us the opportunity to obtain an in-depth understanding of the integration process.

The chief executive officers of each system are owed special appreciation for agreeing to participate in and fund the study. These include Richard Risk, Advocate Health Care; Boone Powell Jr., Baylor Health Care System; Richard A. Norling, Fairview Hospital and Healthcare Services; Ronald R. Aldrich, Franciscan Health System; Gail L. Warden, Henry Ford Health System; Judith C. Pelham, Mercy Health Services; David L. Bernd, Sentara Health System; Glenn R. Mitchell, formerly of Sentara Health System; Peter K. Ellsworth, Sharp HealthCare; Donald A. Brennan, formerly of Sisters of Providence; Sister Dona Taylor, Sisters of Providence; Pat Hays, formerly of Sutter Health; Van Johnson, Sutter Health; Terry Hartshorn, UniHealth; and Paul Teslow, formerly of UniHealth. Their candid and lively discussions at the semiannual CEO meetings provided perhaps the most enriching insights of the entire study.

A second set of people from the participating systems, who became known affectionately as the Research Advisory Group

(RAG), were the system workhorses. They (and their staffs) provided the key system contacts for the study, reviewed the study instruments, and oversaw the many data collection efforts. Their willingness to commit their resources made the study possible; their experience-driven insights kept it on course. Members of the Research Advisory Group include Charles Francis, Advocate Health Care; Joel T. Allison, Baylor Health Care System; L. Gerald Bryant, Baylor Health Care System; Al Swinney, Baylor Health Care System; Bonnie Marsh, Fairview Hospital and Healthcare Services; Pamela Tibbetts, Fairview Hospital and Healthcare Services; Ellen Barron, Franciscan Health System; Vinod K. Sahney, Ph.D., Henry Ford Health System; Peter W. Butler, Henry Ford Health System; Peter Mannix, Mercy Health Services; Ken Rice, Sentara Health System; Jan Cetti, Sharp HealthCare; Peter Bigelow, Sisters of Providence; John P. Lee, Sisters of Providence–Oregon; William L. Dowling, Ph.D., formerly of Sisters of Providence; Mark Parrington, formerly of Sutter Health; and Dennis W. Strum, Ph.D., UniHealth. We are also grateful to Nancy Donaldson and Alberta Pedroja at UniHealth for their assistance in preparing the clinical integration case study in Chapter Six, to Bill Arnold at Franciscan Health System West for his assistance in preparing the functional integration case study in Chapter Four, and to Pat Fry at Sutter Health for his assistance in preparing the governance and management case study in Chapter Seven.

Also crucial to the study were the system clinical representatives, including Michael Soper, M.D., Advocate Health Care; John F. Anderson, M.D., and Charles Jarrett, M.D., Baylor University Medical Center; Gordy Alexander, M.D., and Robert Meiches, M.D., Fairview Hospital and Healthcare Services; Greg Semerdjian, M.D., Franciscan Health System–West; William Conway, M.D., Henry Ford Health System; Bruce L. Van Cleave, M.D., Mercy Health Services; Stuart Baker, M.D., and Robert Brickman, M.D., Sentara Health System; and William J. Kane, M.D., formerly of Sharp HealthCare. These people opened doors to the clinical arena, giving us access to many people and places that might otherwise have been closed to us. Their contributions were particularly valuable as we examined clinical integration issues in greater depth during the fourth year of the study.

A special thanks is due to Walter J. McNerney, M.H.A., Herman Smith Professor of Health Policy, Northwestern University, for his role as facilitator and provocateur at the semiannual CEO meetings. His ability to direct discussions and ask insightful questions resulted in meetings in which everyone felt as if they had acquired a year's worth of knowledge in two days.

Many research associates, research assistants, and support staff members worked on the study over the years. Special appreciation and recognition is due Alice D. Schaller, who oversaw all aspects of manuscript preparation. Cindy Tenny, Lisa Roehl, and Greg Evans, all of Northwestern University, and Kim Doggett, Joan Iverson, and Diane Kiffin of KPMG provided important support. Special recognition is due those who provided research assistance throughout the study: Susan Buettner, Annice Cody, Kelly Devers, Stephen Hiscott, Michael Huff, Kathleen Hull, Elizabeth Lock, Craig Pederson, Juliana Shortell, Tony Simons, Simon Singh, Michelle Snyder, and Tom Vonk. Stephen Hiscott, Kathleen Hull, and Michelle Snyder helped prepare several of the case studies used in the book. Special acknowledgement is due Linda Lin and Shenglin Wang for their computer work on the project.

Many colleagues provided assistance during the study. Linda Cape of KPMG and Mary Kay Donald, formerly of KPMG, and Edward F. X. Hughes, M.D., Joel Shalowitz, M.D., and Frank Lefevre, M.D., of Northwestern University, participated in many of the study site visits. Thomas R. Prince provided critical financial data and insights. David S. Dranove conducted important analyses to further the understanding of key study issues.

The book has also benefited from the superb work of the Jossey-Bass team led by Becky McGovern and from the suggestions of several outside reviewers. Walter Zelman, formerly of the Agency for

Health Care Policy and Research, provided many valuable comments and insights on Chapter Eight regarding public policy implications.

We are also deeply grateful to Johnson & Johnson for their support during the final year. Their generosity allowed us to examine clinical integration issues in greater depth than would have otherwise been possible.

S.M.S.

R.R.G.

D.A.A.

K.M.E.

J.B.M.

The Authors

Stephen M. Shortell, Ph.D., is the A. C. Buehler Distinguished Professor of Health Services Management and professor of organization behavior in the Department of Organization Behavior at the J. L. Kellogg Graduate School of Management, Northwestern University. Dr. Shortell also holds appointments in the Department of Sociology and the Department of Community Medicine, School of Medicine at Northwestern and is a member of the Institute for Health Services Research and Policy Studies. He is an elected member of the Institute of Medicine of the National Academy of Sciences, has served as president of the Association for Health Services Research, and is a past chairman of the Accrediting Commission for Graduate Education in Health Services Administration.

Dr. Shortell received his undergraduate degree from the University of Notre Dame, his master's degree in public health and hospital administration from UCLA, and his Ph.D. in the behavioral sciences from the University of Chicago.

A leading health care scholar, Dr. Shortell is the recipient of many awards, including the distinguished Baxter Prize for innovative health services research. He and his colleagues have also received the George R. Terry Book of the Year Award from the Academy of Management, the James R. Hamilton Book of the Year Award from the American College of Healthcare Executives, and several article of the year awards from the American College of Healthcare Executives and the National Institute for Health Care Management.

Robin R. Gillies, Ph.D., is a research assistant professor at the Institute for Health Services Research and Policy Studies, Northwestern University, and the project director of the Health Systems Integration Study.

Dr. Gillies received her undergraduate degree in political science from the University of California, Irvine, and her master's and Ph.D. in political science from Northwestern University. Her background includes teaching, research, and administration. She was project director of the Intensive Care Unit Research Project at Northwestern University, with Dr. Stephen Shortell as the principal investigator, which investigated the organization and performance of intensive care units. She is also working with Dr. Shortell on a study of the implementation and impact of continuous quality improvement/total quality management on U.S. health care organizations.

David A. Anderson is the partner in charge of KPMG Peat Marwick's National Health Systems Integration Practice. He was formerly partner in charge of the Health Care Consulting Practice for the firm's central region and partner in charge of consulting for the firm's Minneapolis office.

Mr. Anderson received his undergraduate degree from the University of South Dakota and his M.B.A. from the University of Iowa. He is a member of the American Institute of Certified Public Accountants. Mr. Anderson has a wide range of experience working with regional health systems and hospitals throughout the United States on strategic financial and capital planning; mergers, acquisitions, and divestitures; organizational and financial feasibility studies; and shared risk analysis and corporate and management repositioning analysis.

Karen Morgan Erickson is a manager with KPMG Peat Marwick's National Health Care Strategy Practice, and she served as an engagement manager for the Health Systems Integration Study. Ms. Erickson specializes in strategy development for a wide array of health care clients (for example, health systems, academic medical centers, multispecialty group practices, community hospitals in both rural and urban areas, and physician-hospital organizations). In particular, she has experience in strategic planning, mergers and acquisitions, multiunit system integration, and service line planning.

Ms. Erickson received her undergraduate degree in biology from St. Olaf College and holds a master's degree in hospital and health care administration from the University of Minnesota. She held administrative positions at a major academic medical center, a community hospital, and a multispecialty group practice before joining KPMG Peat Marwick.

John B. Mitchell is a principal in KPMG Peat Marwick's National Health Care Strategy Practice, and he served as an engagement manager for the Health Systems Integration Study. He specializes in providing services to health care and medical technology industry clients in the areas of strategic planning, mergers and acquisitions, multiunit system integration and effectiveness, and service line planning.

Mr. Mitchell received his B.S. degree in industrial administration and economics from Iowa State and graduated from the University of Minnesota with a J.D. degree and a master's degree in hospital and health care administration. Prior to joining Peat Marwick, Mr. Mitchell worked in the acquisitions and development department of a large not-for-profit multihospital system. He has also held positions in the legal department of an academic medical center and in the health law department of a Minneapolis law firm.

Remaking Health Care
in America

1

Beyond Fragmentation
Building a Community of Care

Toto, I don't think we are in Kansas anymore.
Dorothy, The Wizard of Oz

The U.S. health care system is unnecessarily fragmented, over-specialized, and unable to respond to rapid change. It is very good at suboptimization, but one would hesitate to claim that as a *core competence*. It is also very good at conducting professional "turf wars," but few would wish to consider that a *core capability*. The core competencies and capabilities of the U.S. health care system (aside from its marvelous technology) are largely yet to be developed because they require reaching beyond individual jobs, careers, professions, groups, departments, divisions, and organizational boundaries. This will be a long, arduous journey marked by honest differences about both what to do and how to do it. The journey is presently made much more difficult by the lack of a common set of financial incentives that would link insurers, payers, providers, and patients, and by the lack of a clearly articulated national health policy. For that matter, we do not even share a collective vision of what we want the U.S. health system to be.

Perhaps the central feature of the U.S. health care system is *fragmentation*. Fragmentation exists at multiple levels. The most obvious is at the level of direct patient care, where many patients engage multiple providers across different settings, each provider asking questions that the patient thought were answered at the initial point of contact with the system. But the fragmentation the patient faces is, of course, the direct result of highly specialized providers operating within highly complex organizational structures. The providers and the organizations with which they are affiliated are, in turn, driven by conflicting financial incentives and public policy. For example, fee-for-service, per diem, and capitation payment arrangements create different incentives for providers regarding use of resources. From a public policy perspective, the lack of a basic benefit package for all Americans results in thousands of different policies and coverages while still leaving approximately forty-three million Americans without any insurance. Fragmented policy and payment combined with fragmented providers and complex organizational structures inevitably result in fragmented patient care delivery. This fragmentation is very costly, currently running at approximately 15 percent of the country's gross national product and over one trillion dollars. Until recently, however, it is the price we have been willing to pay to maintain the cherished American values of autonomy, individuality, self-determination, and diversity.

Health care reform will not succeed until we seriously challenge some of these core values. To what degree should autonomy be pursued at the expense of solidarity? To what extent should individuality be upheld at the neglect of the common good? To what extent shall we cherish self-determination while ignoring the development of a sense of other-directedness? To what extent does an emphasis on diversity threaten a sense of community? To what extent do we continue to support fragmentation and specialization as opposed to integration and a sense of wholeness? These are difficult questions faced by all nations and cultures (Hofstede, 1991). But we must understand that these questions represent a continuum of choices rather than a demand for simple either/or responses. We are not calling for an end to autonomy, individuality, self-determination, or diversity but rather for an increase in solidarity, greater attention to the common good, promotion of other-directedness, and development of community.

The issue is one of *balance*. The U.S. health care system is *out of balance*. The values underlying the system are not in harmony with each other, resulting in mass suboptimization and frustration (reflected most recently in the 1994 abortive attempt at health reform).

The solution for some is radical reform, perhaps best represented by the single-payer approach. Others favor an incremental approach, such as extending coverage to children, eliminating prior condition restrictions, and channeling more Medicare and Medicaid patients into HMOs. But in either case (and in myriad variations in between), an accepted vision of the U.S. health care system is lacking, although several have been proposed (see, for example, Institute for Alternative Futures, 1992). There is no overall framework of what we would like to accomplish as a nation regardless of whether implementation is radical or incremental. Although the U.S. Public Health Service's year 2000 goals (Institute of Medicine, 1990) provide some objectives, they have not been systematically linked or integrated into any of the most recent health care reform proposals. Some who favor more radical reform might well accept more incremental reform if they could see what it was leading to, if they could see it as part of an overall plan as opposed to individual pieces of legislation that attempt to satisfy the most vocal interest groups (at least temporarily). Similarly, those who favor more incremental reform might at least better understand those advocating more radical reform if the latter's arguments were better grounded in dealing with the complexity of the U.S. health system. Many view radical reform as a knee-jerk copycat response based on the experience of other nations, particularly Canada.

The differing viewpoints involve both the *scope* and *speed* of change, as outlined in Figure 1.1.

When the speed of change is fast but the scope is relatively narrow, we have targeted experimentation. Examples include some state health reform efforts, such as those occurring or attempted in Florida, Minnesota, Oregon, and Washington. Viewed from a national perspective, these efforts involve only a small portion of

Figure 1.1. Assessing Approaches to Change.

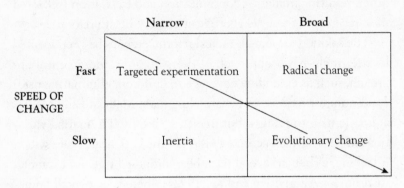

SCOPE OF CHANGE

	Narrow	Broad
Fast	Targeted experimentation	Radical change
Slow	Inertia	Evolutionary change

SPEED OF CHANGE

the country and are in various stages of debate and implementation. However, from the perspective of the states themselves, these efforts could well be viewed as radical change. As shown in Figure 1.1, radical change involves rapid change across a broad scope of activities. Most Americans perceived the Clinton Health Care Security Proposal (the Health Security Act of 1994) as "too much, too soon." As a result, many policy analysts are advocating evolutionary, incremental change in which the eventual scope of change may indeed be broad (involving a more comprehensive benefit package that covers more Americans with new sets of payers and accountability mechanisms) but where the pace of implementation is slower, incremental, and sequential. The lower left cell depicts inertia: slow change aimed at a narrow scope of objectives and activities. At present, it appears that we are pursuing the diagonal arrow of targeted experimentation that we hope will lead to evolutionary change over time. We appear to have largely rejected both the radical and status quo approaches, although a vocal minority can still be found in both cells.

A large part of the challenge in deciding on the speed and scope of change involves the enormous size, complexity, and diversity of the United States. Whatever may be decided at the national or state levels must ultimately be implemented locally. Health care is ultimately a "local business." While the problems of fragmentation, overspecialization, suboptimization, and inability to change rapidly must be worked on simultaneously at multiple levels of society, the implications and consequences are perhaps best revealed at the local community level. Ultimately, the challenge of health care reform is the challenge of *building community*.

Building community is difficult. While modern technology has made it possible for people to be physically closer to each other, other forces such as increased ethnic diversity and social class differences increase psychological distance. Although it would be nice to eliminate the root causes of such separateness (by eliminating poverty, for example), more pragmatically "community" must be built given the hand that has been dealt. This must be done by working across ethnic, educational, geographic, and social class boundaries, to say nothing of organizational and professional boundaries.

There are at least five building blocks to developing community (Peck, 1987). The first is that people must be given or provide for themselves a reason to reach out. This requires an *overarching vision* that links the interests of all parties. Such a vision provides everyone with something for himself or herself that can only be achieved through working with others.

The second building block is to encourage a *psychology of abundance*. This involves looking for win/win situations, using creative approaches to expand resources and rewards for all rather than viewing decisions from a win/lose perspective.

The third building block is to develop the *capability for vulnerability*. Individuals, groups, and organizations need to honestly and with understanding recognize each other's shortcomings. In such recognition lies the opportunity for collaboration. Health care professionals and the organizations with which they are affiliated have a great problem with vulnerability because of their involvement in the sham of perfectionism. Perfectionism does not tolerate error or acknowledge mistakes because this lessens one's image among peers as a technically proficient caregiver. Denial and blaming replaces *learning* from mistakes.

The fourth building block is to create opportunities to *learn from each other*. Those involved in community-building must create laboratories for learning and develop reservoirs of shared experience.

The fifth building block is to develop a cadre of leaders and a *depth of leadership*. Peck (1987, p. 72), for example, has stated that an essential aspect of community is that it is "a group of all leaders." But effective leaders are also good followers as each contributes his or her comparative advantage to the community at large.

The challenge is that these building blocks never stay in place! The work of community-building must be renewed each day in an endless process. Tensions and setbacks will arise regarding issues of size, structure, authority, inclusivity, intensity, commitment, individuality, task definition, and ritual (Peck, 1987). Overly large organizations are not conducive to community-building. How do we make our health care organizations smaller? Structures that are not aligned with changing strategies frustrate people when they attempt to "work against the system." Authority arguments over who is in charge turn our heads inward, away from the needs of patients and the community. Framing decisions around who is in and who is out (that is, inclusivity versus exclusivity) does not build community. Individuals and groups will differ in their intensity and commitment to the community's mission, goals, and objectives. As previously noted, a preoccupation with individuality mitigates against developing a sense of solidarity. Tasks are frequently viewed differently if they become the battleground for protection of turf and advancement of one's professional identity. Finally, health professionals have differing rituals and customs that can serve to divide one group from another.

"Building community" served as the basis for the development of much of sociological theory in the eighteenth and nineteenth centuries. As we head toward the twenty-first century, there appears to be renewed interest in refocusing on the community (see, for example, American Hospital Association, 1993b; Healthcare Forum, 1993; Institute for Health Care Improvement, 1994; and Sigmond, 1995). Some of this interest is driven by the historical community origins of many health care organizations, some by the newly emerging capitation-based payment arrangements emphasizing responsibility for "enrolled lives" (Enthoven, 1993), and some by the recognition of the need for community population-based planning regardless of source or type of payment. In response, a variety of health care organizations—hospitals, physician groups, health plans, home health agencies, hospices, skilled nursing facilities, and others—are joining together to form organized or integrated health systems with the intent of delivering a broad array of services across the continuum of care in a cost-effective fashion. We formally define an *organized delivery system* as a network of organizations that provides or arranges to provide a coordinated continuum of services to a defined population and is willing to be held clinically and fiscally accountable for the outcomes and the health status of the population served (Shortell, Gillies, and others, 1993). This definition underscores the fact that organized delivery systems may be built through "virtual" integration processes encompassing contracts and strategic alliances as well as through direct ownership (Goldsmith, 1994). It is also important to recognize that there are many models of organized delivery systems, including those built around former multihospital systems (for example, Intermountain Health Care); those built around physician groups (for example, Mayo Clinic); those built around insurance companies (for example, Aetna, Cigna, and Prudential); and other hybrid models representing various combinations of the above (for example, Allina, Kaiser-Permanente, and Cigna-Lovelace Clinic). The systems examined in this book are rapidly evolving toward the hybrid model, but most have their historical roots in multihospital systems.

A central challenge that such organized delivery systems face, however, is to go beyond being organized or integrated delivery systems as legal entities or in press releases and to actually deliver and manage more coordinated clinical care that truly adds value to patients. Further, these systems must reach *beyond patients* to enhance the health status of the *communities* they serve. In this respect, organized delivery systems become the building blocks for creating *community health care management systems*, a concept developed further in Chapter Two. To be effective, health systems must do a better job of building the "internal community" in order to serve the external community. In many respects, this book is about building internal community—a community of caregivers and caregiving processes that enhances the health both of individuals and the larger community within which they live.

This involves linking the organized delivery system concept to the notion of community health and well-being. Organized delivery systems are social and organizational mechanisms for improving community health and well-being through disease prevention and health promotion, illness treatment, rehabilitation, chronic disease management, and provision of palliative care. These responsibilities are carried out in *collaboration* with community health and social service agencies (Bader, 1994) as part of an overall community health care management system. This idea is not new. What is new is that market forces are now pushing toward a union of the personal and public health systems to reinforce the long-held views of health planners and public health professionals. Many communities have assembled the pieces. The challenge now is to get them to work together. But this requires a vision of what we want the system to do. What do we want community health to be? What should organized delivery systems designed to achieve these objectives look like? What is a community health care management system? We address these questions in Chapter Two.

2

Working Toward an Ideal System

Some time ago, one of the authors overheard the following conversation in the waiting room of an ambulatory care clinic. Speaking to the receptionist, a patient made the following comment (expressed in a tone of slight exasperation):

> You know, I have a pretty simple wish. I want to stay healthy and productive. When I become sick I want to get well as quickly as possible. But I know that costs are also important. So I want to know what's done to me is really needed and is done as efficiently as possible. Do you think that's too much to ask for?

We can ask for anything, but it doesn't mean we are going to get it. This patient was a well-educated, reasonably sophisticated and motivated consumer of health services. But not everyone is. For example, while few individuals desire to be sick, many are unwilling to make the necessary investment to remain well. The health care system deals with a tremendous variety in patients' genetic stock as well as their ability and willingness to enhance, maintain, and restore their health. This diversity presents challenging organizational problems.

"I want to know that what is done to me is really needed. . . ." But medicine is both an art and a science. Physicians and other members

of the health care team often don't know what is really needed. It has been estimated that as much as 70 percent of medical treatment is provided without a firm scientific basis (Williamson, 1991) even though the best medical judgment and clinical experience are being used.

"And is done as efficiently as possible." There are currently great pressures to contain costs, improve productivity, and increase efficiency. The challenge lies in achieving efficiency not just for an individual at a single point in time but across a group of patients over time. What may not seem efficient for an individual patient may be efficient on average for a group of patients; for example, block scheduling of patient appointments. The challenge is one of *mass customization* (Davis, 1987; Kotha, 1995); that is, establishing procedures and processes that apply to most patients while building in flexibility to adapt to the idiosyncratic needs of each individual.

The Ideal Health System: The Patient's Perspective

So what might an ideal health system look like to a patient? The following two scenarios, one real and one fictitious, introduce us to some of the elements of an ideal system.

Scenario I

On August 13, 1994, Robert Morris, CEO of Laurel Health System in Wellsboro, Pennsylvania, was involved in a serious motorcycle accident that left him with multiple fractures, a collapsed lung, and related injuries. We pick up Mr. Morris' story shortly after surgery.

> As Morris began showing signs of improvement . . . the demand for trauma beds required his transfer to a general intensive care unit (ICU). What Egan [trauma nurse Liz Egan] did in response deeply impressed the 44 year old Morris, who knows about the workings of hospitals through his experience as a hospital CEO.

Egan not only accompanied Morris to the ICU but stayed there to brief the staff on the nuances of his condition. She even returned several times to check up on him. As Morris traveled the inpatient continuum from the ICU to a trauma transition unit leading up to his discharge four days after the accident, Egan visited him twice more.

"My condition was apparently more precarious than I was aware of, and Liz wanted to make sure that nothing fell through the cracks with me," says Morris. "I was impressed by what she did, either by the hospital's design or on her own to maintain continuity of care. Surrounded by all of that wonder whiz-bang technology and clinical ability, her concern for me made the difference."

You see Liz Egan–style behavior all the time in health care. It's what Morris calls an "other centered" approach that he's attempted to foster across the many sites and services that make up Laurel Health System. It's the smooth hand off from one care giver to the next, the connections between services, the communication that ensures a smooth transition: seamless care.

Many hospitals do this well within their own walls, as patients traverse from one unit to the next, and many segments that make up the continuum do so individually—from ambulatory clinics to physicians' offices to home health to hospice. But as integrated health systems evolve and push into their communities to provide total care for defined populations, the passing of the baton from one care setting to the next becomes more important—and much easier said than done.

It is the smooth functioning of the continuum of care that separates real health systems from loose alliances of providers. A well coordinated continuum adds value to a system's performance. [Lumsdon, 1994, p. 28]

Scenario II

Mr. Dwight Taylor is a fictitious patient featured in the *Henry Ford Health System 1994 System Report*. His story is told below.

> I remembered telling my friend Fred at lunch that I had awakened with a terrible headache. I had ended rushing to work and still missed a conference call. Then Fred started laughing and said, "Dwight, you are losing it, you are drooling."
>
> I reached for a napkin to wipe my mouth, but I couldn't get it to my mouth. Something was wrong. My hand couldn't grab the napkin, and it felt heavy. I was feeling very strange. Fred looked blurred, out of focus. My left arm was tingling, and my speech was slurred. I thought "I am having a heart attack." After that, I remember that Fred was yelling for someone to call 911. . . . I ended up in an ambulance then a hospital emergency room. Later, I found out it was Henry Ford Hospital in Detroit. . . .
>
> When I [next] woke up, standing over me was a man in a white coat who introduced himself as Dr. Steven Levine, a neurologist at Henry Ford. I remembered him from the emergency room. He said the stroke I had was a moderate one. He tried to assure me but said he still needed to do some more tests to figure out why I had a stroke.
>
> Dr. Levine said that because I was a Henry Ford patient, he had been able to call up my medical history on the computer in the emergency room the night before. He had also talked with my family physician, Dr. Dickenson, about my condition. Dr. Levine noted that I'd been a heavy smoker for some 25 years. . . .
>
> Dr. Levine told me that I need speech and occupational therapy. He talked with Dr. Dickenson again who

Dr. Levine said would oversee the rest of my care. He arranged for me to have my rehab at Henry Ford's Cottage Hospital in Grosse Pointe Farms, which is across the road from Dr. Dickenson's office and not far from my house.

Rehab took several months, but after only about six weeks, I was able to go back to work part time. That made me feel better knowing I could still support my family and do my job. (p. 8)

As an accompanying note to Dwight Taylor's saga, Henry Ford's brochure notes that "the Taylors have ready access to the full range of services that 'an integrated' health care system provides—coordination of referrals, a life long medical history and continuum of care, a common patient log and ready access to primary care, specialty and support services at a network of convenient locations. . . . The system also offers the advantages of test results being shared, not repeated. And care provided at one site can be reviewed electronically at another site, upon the patient's transfer or referral" (Henry Ford Health System, 1994, p. 6).

These two scenarios illustrate the importance of *caring, communication*, and *information* in providing coordinated continuous patient care. In Mr. Morris' case, the caring, communication, and information transfer appeared to depend primarily on the commitment and competence of Liz Egan. What might have happened if there had been no Liz Egan? In Mr. Taylor's situation, the caring, communication, and information seem to be more institutionalized or "integrated" within the Henry Ford Health System's practices, policies, and procedures. And yet one knows that how things are described in a glossy annual report are not always how they appear in practice for each individual patient. The hallmark of an excellent health system is its ability to *consistently* provide well-coordinated, continuous care that produces desired outcomes for each and every patient day in and day out.

The Ideal Health System: The Health Care Executive's Perspective

The daydream of an ideal system—and the harsh reality—are illustrated below by Mr. John Smythe, CEO of the fictitious General Health System (Voluntary Hospitals of America, 1994).

The Daydream

The board meeting ended 15 minutes early, and John decided to spend a few quiet minutes in the solitude of his office before going home. As he walked to his office, he thought about how unusually harmonious his day had been. No, it was just this day that was unusual—the whole situation seemed too perfect to be real. "I used to only be concerned with the operations of my hospital" he marveled.

Now John ran a large regional delivery system with myriad highly evolved characteristics:

- Focused on meeting the needs of a specific population

- Offering facilities and service capacity exactly matched to the needs of the population

- Managed not by controls or incentives, but rather, through a strong, positive culture

- Allowing physicians to practice collegially without worrying about the business side of their practices. Clinicians collectively determined the most appropriate clinical pathways to follow for each disease and/or condition.

- Accessible and responsive to the purchasers of care in the community for delivering quality of service, value, and cost-effectiveness

- Supported by integrated information technology linking various clinicians and distant locations,

supplying information for reviewing clinical
approaches, monitoring outcomes of procedures
and patterns of care, and placing the most recent
and advanced clinical knowledge in the hands of
the clinician at the point of care

- Endowed with sufficient capital to meet investment
  needs and allocate resources in a system-wide (not
  entity-specific) manner.

- Consistently managing care across the care continuum with a long-term focus

- Positioned where financial incentives are aligned
  through the entire delivery system to meet the needs
  of purchasers

The Harsh Reality

As John opened the door to his now dark office, he was
jolted by a loud pounding. Were the decorators still at
work at this late hour? . . .

"This meeting will come back to order." John Smythe,
CEO of the City General Hospital, shuddered, quickly
shook his head and realized that he had been dream-
ing. . . .The hospital's Medical Executive Committee was
being called back to order after a short break. It was time
to continue discussing how the hospital and physicians
could work together to meet the challenge of new managed care plans. The local HMO wanted to begin capi-
tating primary care physicians and put the hospital at
risk for length of stay.

John looked around the room and realized how far
from reality his short daydream into a future fantasy
world had taken him. The advanced concepts needed for
advanced provider integration seemed irrelevant to his
organization in its current state. His head was swimming:

- Managed care? We haven't begun to learn to live with the small amounts of insurance risk involved in our holdbacks for the local HMO.

- Collegial medical practice? The physicians are in 300 separate small groups, each claiming to practice the highest quality medicine possible. There is no discussion among physicians about appropriateness of anything they do in their own individual offices.

- Align incentives? Each physician is thinking about his or her own practice economics—and each physician/hospital/HMO issue is always framed in a defined-sum manner.

- Balanced capacity? My people are trying to figure out how to fill more beds!

- Work in a capitated framework? We're still arguing about the appropriate discount from charges the surgical specialists need to give the PHO.

- Advanced information systems? We can't even supply encounter data to understand from a transactional standpoint what our overall utilization experience has been.

- Improved health status? We haven't even measured the current health indicators in our community, let alone our impact on the community's health.

Suddenly John realized the enormity of the task in front of him. None of the current paradigms, working relationships, organizational and management structures, payment mechanisms, etc. were sufficient to even begin working within the new health care environment and its challenges—managed care, accountability for cost and quality, and the need for integration.

His daydream needed to become a reality. He knew
where he needed to go but not how to begin. "How do I
get there from here?" he cried.

These scenarios introduce almost all of the elements of an ideal
health care system, which are summarized in the list below and are
similar to the four key characteristics of community care networks
that have been put forth by the American Hospital Association
(AHA), namely, having a community health focus, providing a
seamless continuum of care, managing within fixed resources, and
being accountable to the community (American Hospital Association, 1993b).

Key Elements of an Ideal Health Care System

- Focuses on meeting the population's health needs

- Matches service capacity to meet the population's needs

- Coordinates and integrates care across the continuum

- Has information systems to link patients, providers,
  and payers across the continuum of care

- Is able to provide information on cost, quality outcomes, and patient satisfaction to multiple stakeholders—patients, employees, staff, payers and purchasers,
  community groups, and external review bodies

- Uses financial incentives and organizational structure
  to align governance, management, physicians, and
  other caregivers in support of achieving shared
  objectives

- Is able to continuously improve the care that it provides

- Is willing and able to work with others to ensure that
  the community's health objectives are met

What we as patients want from a health care system are:

- Providers knowledgeable about our health history—allergies, family/genetic predisposition to illness, life-style, history, and so on.

- Up-to-date information on health maintenance and improvement, disease prevention, and cost-effective treatment innovations *before* we might need them.

- Convenient access when we do need care.

- Excellent treatment from people who work well together.

- Polite, courteous attention, and having our questions answered.

- Appropriate and coordinated follow-up care.

- Smooth handoffs from one provider to another and one treatment setting to another as appropriate. We don't want to have to repeat the same answers or provide the same information.

- To be informed of changes in the organization and its providers *ahead of time*.

- An organization that can learn from its mistakes. Errors and mistakes are inevitable (Leape, 1994), but providers and organizations should not make the same mistake twice. They should continuously get better over time.

This is a tall order, but if we expect no less from organizations that make our television sets, digital pagers, cellular phones, and automobiles, why should we expect less from those that provide our health and medical services?

The primary challenge is to overcome the fragmentation discussed in Chapter One. The culprits include imperfect information,
incomplete communication, conflicting incentives, and organizational and professional biases (Institute for the Future, 1993a). In
order to counteract these influences, an integrated system needs to
create a team-oriented culture, develop flexible organizational structures, invest in information systems, and offer relevant incentives.
But the question remains: how do we get there from here?

The Community Health Care Management System

Based on four years of research involving eleven organized delivery
systems across the United States, we believe a starting point is to
develop a *community health care management system*, as shown in
Figure 2.1.

The system begins with knowing its current and future "customers" and the communities in which they reside. We refer to this
as *community/population-based health needs assessment*. This involves
defining the specific segments of the population and the geographic
area that the system wishes to serve. This will be determined by the
system's mission and values and by the configuration of other health
providers, systems, and resources in the community relative to the
populations of interest. It will also be influenced by the system's perceived capabilities relative to those of others. These populations are
likely to include individuals both with and without health insurance coverage. Those with insurance can be broken out by whether
they are an "enrolled life," either the system's own managed care
product or a contracted managed care product. Those without insurance coverage and special populations (for example, children on
Medicaid) can be broken out by geography, education, income, and
ethnic characteristics, among others. What is important is to project the needs of the different groups and convert these into likely
utilization of health care services and resources. To the extent that
capitated payment or prepayment of some form continues to grow

Figure 2.1. The Community Health Care Management System.

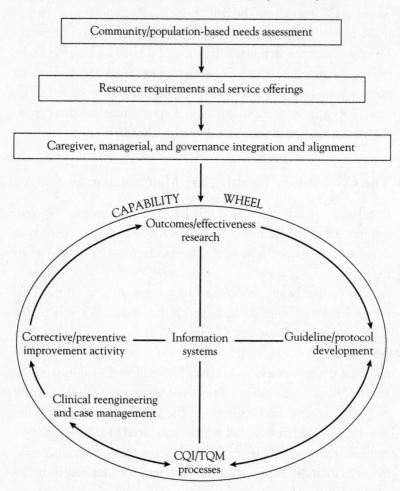

Source: Shortell, Gillies, and Devers, 1995, p. 151. This figure first appeared in
The Milbank Quarterly.

throughout the country, health systems have an incentive to take a more assertive and activist stance toward maintaining and promoting the health of the population they serve. This incentive will also require a system to take a *broader* perspective of what contributes to good health and, therefore, become more involved in issues that influence community health such as crime, alcohol and substance abuse, and domestic violence.

This requires systems to go beyond traditional data collection and analysis. For example, the Hospital Association of Pennsylvania has developed a five-phase model of assessment: (1) developing a county health profile that "blends" data from multiple sources, including small-area variation analysis of clinical practice patterns; (2) collecting original data on personal health behaviors combined with a community health resource inventory profile and a health care economic impact statement; (3) sharing information from the preceding two phases with a series of focus groups comprising individuals likely to be affected by the decisions made; (4) developing a community action plan based on all of the above input; and (5) monitoring the implementation and evaluating the impact as actions unfold (Hospital Association of Pennsylvania, 1993). The Crozer-Keystone Health System in Media, Pennsylvania, has used many components of this model and, in the process, has directly linked top management compensation to achievement of selected community health objectives, such as immunization rates and provision of prenatal care in the first trimester (Gardner, 1994). Allina, an evolving insurer-provider integrated system based in Minneapolis–St. Paul has used health status needs assessment to develop such explicit objectives as (1) to increase from 75 percent to 95 percent the number of children in the system who are fully immunized for childhood diseases by age 2; (2) to reduce by 50 percent the incidence of breast cancer that reaches an advanced stage before being detected; and (3) to increase early detection of adult-onset diabetes by screening 90 percent of high-risk members

(Voluntary Hospitals of America, 1994). Such objectives are targeted only to Allina's enrolled population and membership and, thus, ignore the larger Minneapolis–St. Paul community. Allina's plans, objectives, and data need to be coordinated with those of other organized delivery systems in the area in order to achieve maximum community-wide impact.

Based on community/population-based health needs assessment, systems can determine the resources and services to offer. The system must be "right sized" to meet the selected population's anticipated needs. This involves determining the number and location of primary care providers, specialists, acute care beds, rehabilitation beds, long-term care beds, home health services, hospice services, and the like. The system must make decisions involving the breadth and depth of services it will offer (Shortell, Gillies, and others, 1993). *Breadth* refers to the number of different services provided across the continuum of care to serve the populations of interest. For example, a system that provides thirty-five different services ranging from primary care to acute care to rehabilitative care has more breadth than one that offers only twenty-five services that may be more narrowly focused on acute care. *Depth* refers to the extent to which a given service is provided at multiple locations or operating units within a system. For example, a system that offers psychiatric care at five of its operating units has more depth (in that service line) than a similarly sized system that offers it at only three locations. As systems across the country examine the breadth and depth of services needed by the community, many find that they have up to 50 percent more specialists, approximately 25 percent less primary care capacity, and up to 50 percent more acute care beds than needed. This is understandable given that the "dominant logic" (Prahalad and Bettis, 1986; Bettis and Prahalad, 1995) of U.S. health care has until recently been the provision of acute illness–oriented inpatient care. But a new dominant logic based on disease prevention, health promotion, and primary care is emerging, resulting in a significant amount of restructuring activity. Just as IBM, the big three American automobile companies, and the airlines have had to relearn their business and construct new "dominant logics," so it is that U.S. health care organizations must do the same.

As shown in Figure 2.1, once the resource requirements and service offerings are determined as a function of the community/ population-based health status assessment, the system faces the challenge of aligning its caregiver, management, and governance structures. *Alignment* means that those who actually deliver health and medical services (caregivers), those who manage them (managers), and those who oversee the process and are accountable to the community (governing boards) are working together rather than at cross-purposes with each other. For example, given the pressures for more cost-effective care, physicians, nurses, and other caregivers are having to reorganize themselves into multidisciplinary teams and service lines using treatment protocols, guidelines, pathways, and outcome data to coordinate care across the care continuum. In like fashion, management and governance structures must change to support the new forms of delivering health and medical services. The multidisciplinary provision of care across the continuum will not work if attempted within outmoded management and governance structures. Management structures must be changed to reflect continuum of care and service line responsibilities. Similarly, governance structures must be changed to reflect area-wide responsibilities for the health of defined populations, with greater attention given to achieving systemwide objectives in addition to individual operating-unit objectives. The alignment of caregiver, management, and governance functions is discussed further in Chapter Seven.

Once the population's needs are defined, the system is "right sized," and the clinical, managerial, and governance functions are aligned, the system is ready to "perform." This is represented in Figure 2.1 as a *capability wheel* comprising interrelated processes:

outcomes and effectiveness research, guideline and protocol development, CQI/TQM processes, clinical reengineering, case management, taking corrective and preventive action, and measuring the outcome of these actions. All of these activities are anchored by the information systems depicted in the middle of the wheel.

The underlying logic of the capability wheel is as follows. One first begins with obtaining benchmark data and information on state-of-the-art outcomes and effectiveness for a given condition, procedure, or state of health. This serves as a base for developing the system's own guidelines, protocols, and pathways for managing the health of defined populations. These guidelines, protocols, and pathways both serve as inputs to quality improvement opportunities and solutions and are influenced by the system's CQI/TQM processes. Hence, the double-headed arrow between the two in Figure 2.1. In turn, a system's CQI/TQM processes influence its efforts at clinical reengineering, which is defined as the elimination and/or significant reorganization of fundamental clinical functions. Clinical reengineering and case management also has a reciprocal effect on the system's CQI/TQM processes. Ultimately, corrective and preventive improvement activities are undertaken that in turn result in assessment of the outcomes: what worked, what didn't work, and why. This "local" information and experience feeds back into new developments nationally in an iterative fashion as the wheel turns, continuously measuring and improving the defined populations'(the communities') ability to prevent disease and to maintain and improve its health.

Three points about the community health care management system should be emphasized. The first is that the capability wheel applies to disease prevention, health maintenance, and health promotion activities, as well as to acute and chronic care treatment. In fact, it can be argued that outcomes research, protocol development, CQI/TQM processes, and related activities that are focused more on disease prevention and health maintenance and promotion will have a larger impact and payoff than much of the current focus on acute and chronic care (Rundall and Schauffler, 1995). For example, avoiding one low-birth-weight infant can save between $14,000 and $30,000 in health care costs (Office of Technology Assessment, 1991), and investments in improved prenatal care have been shown to result in cost savings of direct medical care of $3.38 for every $1.00 spent (Institute of Medicine, 1988).

The second point is that, at least in metropolitan areas, no single organized delivery system can develop all components of a community health care management system nor does it have to own all of the components that make up the system. The community health care management system will be composed of *virtual organizations*, networks of organized delivery systems and community agencies willing to share risk, costs, rewards, knowledge, and skills. Most of the study systems have developed significant strategic alliances with other providers and insurers as well as with public health departments and social and community service organizations.

The third point is to emphasize the important integrative role played by information systems. In some respects, this is the least developed aspect of the community health care management system concept. Because of its central role, this underdevelopment slows down achievement of the other components of the system. Study participants are spending tens of millions of dollars to expand and upgrade their information systems so that they can link patients and providers across the continuum of care. But beyond that is the need to incorporate community and public health data and to link one organized delivery system's data with another's. The Community Health Information Networks (CHINS) represent a potentially promising approach to the issue.

The community health care management system concept is consistent with the American Hospital Association's community care network concept (1993), the Hospital Research and Educational Trust's work (1994) on creating community action learning laboratories, the Institute for Health Care Improvement's community collaborative work (1994) involving the application of CQI/TQM principles and processes to community-wide health care problems, and the Healthcare Forum's work (1994) on building healthier communities. The renewed interest in community health care has its historical roots in the landmark report of the Committee on the Cost of Medical Care (1932; Sigmond, 1995). Although there is growing recognition that building healthier communities must extend beyond the efforts of individual organized health care delivery systems, such systems are essential building blocks. To achieve their mission and their potential for community collaboration, these organizations must be infused with the principles of *holography*.

The Holographic Organization

A *hologram* is a photographic plate containing all the information necessary to produce a complete image in each of its parts. When you switch the picture from one part to another, you still see the whole image. The elements required for the whole image are contained within the parts.

The hologram is a powerful metaphor for organizations (Morgan, 1986), systems, and community development. Holographic properties exist at the organizational level to the extent that the organization is represented in each of its constituent parts—divisions, departments, task forces, committees, and individuals. The organization is not merely the sum of its parts but *exists* in each part. This is quite easy to understand in the case of the one-person entrepreneurial firm. In this case, the individual *is* the organization, performing essentially all of the functions associated with product or service development, sales, marketing, accounting, and so on. But as organizations grow large and more complex, they begin to lose their holographic properties: layers of hierarchy, bureaucracy, and specialization emerge. The challenge for large, complex organizations is to regain some of the holographic properties of their youthful beginnings. One way to do this is to become small again by creating smaller organizations within the larger organization. For example, 3M has no division greater than four hundred employees, and Microsoft organizes itself into units of no more than two hundred people each. These companies believe that beyond a certain size, a division or unit will have difficulty sustaining close face-to-face interaction, coordinating activities, and stimulating creative, innovative ideas. Other companies such as Federal Express, Johnson & Johnson, and Xerox attempt to achieve holography by developing a strong culture that unites people across divisions, departments, lines of business, and geography. Organizations also become more holographic when they engage in such activities as training people to perform multiple functions, making greater use of multidisciplinary teams, blurring line and staff responsibilities, providing people with matrix management skills, and developing information systems that facilitate communication among people throughout the organization, thus increasing the opportunities for learning. From the perspective of a patient, as much of the entire health care organization as possible should be embedded or "hard wired" into each person, group, or team that the patient encounters in the process of receiving care.

From an organized delivery system perspective, each operating unit involved in the continuum of care—prevention, primary care, acute care, rehabilitative care, and maintenance care—should have "the system" embedded within it. As discussed in subsequent chapters, this is achieved through functional integration, physician-system integration, and clinical integration. This leads to what we have elsewhere called a sense of "systemness" (Shortell, 1988), in which each unit of the system understands the strategic role it plays within the overall system. In such systems, strategy and structure are viewed as each being embedded within the other like an intertwined rope. For example, a system's vertical integration efforts, its strategic alliances, and its decentralization and empowerment efforts should each be seen as both strategy and structure.

A community health care management system can have holographic properties when the community's overall health and well-being are embedded or contained within each organized delivery system operating in the community. In this way, the organized delivery system's goals and objectives would reflect community-wide goals, and a sense of interdependence would foster collaboration rather than unnecessary competition.

Holographic organizations and systems increase the probability of providing more holistic, coordinated, and continuous cost-effective care to patients and health enhancement services to populations. Holography is the antidote to runaway fragmentation and specialization. At the social and organizational level, *learning* is the key mechanism by which holography operates. Learning is also one of the keys to community-building (see Chapter One). Holographic properties rapidly increase the speed of learning throughout an organization or system, and is the means by which the whole is embedded within each part.

Generating holographic properties is a daunting task because the dysfunctions of fragmentation, needless competition, and reactivity are deeply embedded in our society and culture. Kofman and Senge (1994) suggest that these maladies need to be replaced by what they call "regaining the memory of the whole," recognizing the community nature of the self, and by using language as a creative act (p. 6). They term this transition the Galilean Shift—moving from an emphasis on fragmented parts, individual competition, and reacting to problems, to an emphasis on the whole, on the community, and on creativity (p. 6). Among their suggestions for making this shift is to create experimental and managerial "practice fields" where people can experiment with new approaches for working together, applying skills, and, in our terms, developing holographic properties (p. 22).

To do this, organized delivery systems constituted as holograms will engage continuously in "double loop" learning: questioning the underlying assumptions and dominant logic upon which current practices and policies are based (Argyris, 1982; Senge, 1990). For example, most health systems have assumed that strategic plans should be built around the hospitals within the system, given that hospitals have been the primary generators of capital and the entities with which most physicians were associated through the medical staff organization structure. But some systems are now questioning this underlying assumption as hospitals become less central to the provision of health care services and as physicians join groups and form their own organized entities separate from the hospital. Increasingly, system strategic plans are built around physician groups and primary care networks.

Organized delivery systems with strong holographic properties create more options for themselves—they are no longer psychic prisoners of old paradigms. Such organizations are "clever organizations" (Handy, 1989, p. 15): sharing and pooling resources and knowledge through task forces, creating and executing strategies with the involvement of those closest to the issues, making ongoing use of differentiated structures; they are information based, with great emphasis on continuous learning.

The Role of Integration

Integration is defined as the process by which activities are formed, coordinated, or blended into a functioning or unified whole (Webster's, 1990). Integration is an essential process to building a holographic organization because before the whole can be embedded in each part, it must first exist as a "whole"—that is, something must be brought together from different elements. For example, in order for a hypertensive diabetic patient to receive the same quality care from multispecialty Clinic A within a given system as the patient would from multispecialty Clinic B (that is, for the "whole" to be in each part), the nature of what constitutes high-quality "holistic" hypertensive diabetic care needs to be defined and implemented. This might be done, for example, through the development of guidelines and protocols that stipulate how a variety of steps are to be executed and in what order. Overall case or care management systems would play a similar role. The result is a "whole" that can then be implanted in each part of the system. Thus, integration is both a cause and an effect of a holographic organization. It is a cause in that certain elements, processes, and activities must be coordinated with each other to create "wholes." But integration is also an effect, because as the whole is reflected in each part, the parts give rise to greater integration potential with other parts of the system. A well-integrated part has greater "carrying capacity" to link up and energize other parts of the system and thereby create greater value.

We believe that functional integration, physician-system integration, and clinical integration (Gillies and others, 1993) are the key elements in creating the holographic properties that must exist within an organized delivery system. *Functional integration* is defined as the extent to which key support functions such as financial management, human resources, information systems, strategic planning, and total quality management are coordinated across the operating units of a given system so as to add the greatest overall value to the system. *Physician-system integration* is defined as the extent to which physicians are economically linked to the system, use its facilities and services, and are active participants in its planning, management, and governance. *Clinical integration* is defined as the extent to which patient care services are coordinated across people, functions, activities, processes, and operating units so as to maximize the value of services delivered. Clinical integration includes both horizontal integration (the coordination of activities at the same stage of delivery of care) as well as vertical integration (the coordination of services at different stages)—for example, between acute care and post acute care (Conrad and Dowling, 1990; Fox, 1989).

"Staging" the Ideal System

Building a community health care management system cannot be achieved overnight. Certain key stages or steps must take place before other changes can occur. There needs to be a certain degree of functional integration to assist physician-system integration efforts. In turn, both functional integration and physician-system integration are essential to achieving clinical integration. While putting these steps or building blocks in place can be accelerated (indeed, we argue that they must be accelerated), trying to skip over them altogether results in failure.

The pace and type of integration called for is largely driven by market and external forces. These include the degree of overall managed care penetration in the marketplace, the specific degree of capitated payment that exists, the degree of competition among systems and networks, the activities of major employers and business coalitions, and state health reform legislative initiatives. There exist several classifications of health care market profile stages or phases (American Practice Management, 1993; Coile, 1994; Advisory Board Company, 1993; Voluntary Hospitals of America, 1994). Table 2.1 provides an overview of some of the more important characteristics of each stage; Table 2.2 suggests several delivery system integration activities appropriate to each stage.

As one moves from left to right through the four stages of "market maturity," the components of delivery system integration build on each other. This starts with acquiring the "pieces" of a delivery system and functionally integrating them in the unstructured "access" market stage, and culminates in the need for a high level of clinical integration, associated outcomes reporting, and taking on responsibility for community health status in the "value" market stage.

What Tables 2.1 and 2.2 do not show may be the most important factor in managing the pace of change. This is the amount of *time* before a given market moves from one stage to another. The challenge for those who lead organized delivery systems is to position their systems so that they are only somewhat or "loosely" fit for their current environment while preparing for the newly emerging environment. This is tricky business. The danger in making changes before one has to or in making too large a change is that the market (in other words, the payers) will not yet reward you for it. In the

Table 2.1. Market Stages and Delivery System Organization.

Stage 1 Unstructured "access" market	Stage 2 "Loose cost" market	Stage 3 Consolidated "advanced cost" market	Stage 4 Strict managed care "value" market
• Independent hospitals/ providers • Independent payers • Few HMOs/PPOs • Little managed care penetration— < 20 percent • < 25 percent physicians in groups	• Hospitals/providers begin to merge and forge alliances • Largely independent payers • HMOs/PPOs grow • Managed care penetration grows—20–40 percent • Excess inpatient bed capacity develops • 25–49 percent physicians in groups	• Critical mass of systems/networks emerge • Payers consolidate • Local HMOs/PPOs consolidate and achieve critical mass • Managed care penetration—40–60 percent • Significant inpatient bed reduction • 50–74 percent physicians in groups	• 3–5 systems/networks dominate metropolitan markets • Highly consolidated payer base • Purchaser-provider linkages • Managed care penetration— >60 percent • Capitation payment emerges as a force • 75 percent or more physicians in groups
Example markets Atlanta Little Rock Pittsburgh Savannah	Example markets Chicago Detroit	Example markets Los Angeles Portland Seattle San Francisco	Example markets Albuquerque Minneapolis–St. Paul San Diego

Sources: American Practice Management, 1993; Coile, 1994; Advisory Board Company, 1993; Voluntary Hospitals of America, 1994

Table 2.2. Suggested Level of Delivery System Integration Activity by Market Stage

Stage 1 Unstructured "access" market	Stage 2 "Loose cost" market	Stage 3 Consolidated "advanced cost" market	Stage 4 Strict managed care "value" market
• Acquire the pieces	• Expand functional integration efforts	• Expand physician-system integration efforts	• Expand clinical integration efforts
• Build functional integration	• Accelerate cost-reduction efforts	• Expand risk-based contracting	• Consolidate relationships with insurance partners
• Reduce costs	• Accelerate bed-reduction efforts	• Explore relationships with insurance partners	• Use outcomes data for external accountability and internal quality improvement
• Question the decentralization of capital to operating units	• Develop primary care physician network capacity	• Initiate clinical integration efforts	• Expand population-based planning efforts
• Look for physician and other partners	• Develop other parts of the continuum of care, e.g., home care	• Emphasize disease prevention and health promotion	• Forge stronger partnerships with public health, community, and social service agencies
• Question acute inpatient focus	• Begin physician-system integration efforts	• Establish new management and governance structures	• Take greater responsibility for community health status and well being
	• Begin to consolidate capital development		

process you may also alienate key groups, particularly physicians. The danger of waiting until the market has sufficiently "evolved" is that others may have beaten you to the punch, leaving you with a long, uphill struggle. The secret of success lies in developing what we might call the "Gretzsky Response." When interviewed regarding his phenomenal success as a hockey player, Wayne Gretzsky responded to the effect that other players skate to where the puck is and that he tries to skate to where the puck is going to be. From an organized delivery system's perspective, this requires three skills: (1) the ability to properly assess where the environment is going to be; (2) the ability to assess *how long it will take to get there*; and (3) the ability of the organization to get there either slightly before or at least at the same time that the changes in the environment materialize relative to the competition. In other words, direction, speed, and timing are of the essence.

We believe that most, if not all, communities throughout the United States are moving out of Stage 1 to Stages 2 and 3 with a few advancing to Stage 4 markets. For example, it is estimated that whereas in 1994 36 percent of the United States' population lived in Stage 1 markets, 38 percent in Stage 2 markets, and 24 percent in combined Stage 3 and 4 markets; in 1998 only 6 percent will live in Stage 1 markets, 31 percent in Stage 2 markets, 29 percent in Stage 3 markets, and 34 percent in Stage 4 markets (Johnson & Johnson, 1994).

It is more difficult to assess the speed of change occurring in different communities throughout the country. Based on our experience, however, we believe that the *slowest* part of the transition is going from Stage 1 to Stage 2, due to the considerable inertia exhibited by individual hospitals, fee-for-service payment, and fragmented payers in Stage 1 communities. Once managed care activity is in the neighborhood of 35 to 40 percent penetration (characteristic of Stage 2), the movement to Stage 3 is extremely rapid. Once in Stage 3, the movement to Stage 4 may be somewhat slower than in going from Stage 2 to Stage 3 but not as slow as that from Stage 1 to Stage 2. In Stage 3, the organized delivery system is essentially in a position to accept greater amounts of capitated payment, but the extent to which payers/purchasers are interested in full capitation varies largely as a function of experience in assessing risk. Thus, we envision that Stage 4 markets will exist with various modes and degrees of capitated payment, which in turn will send somewhat mixed signals to organized delivery systems regarding the speed with which they need to continue structuring themselves to care for enrolled populations. As a result, the transition to a Stage 4 delivery system may be somewhat slower. This transition would, of course, be greatly accelerated if national health care reform legislation were passed guaranteeing a set of benefits to all Americans within a range of given premiums that reflect geographic, health status–related, and other adjustments.

What does all of this have to do with creating the ideal health care system as might be reflected in a community health care management system? It is a realistic reminder that creating such a system is a *journey*. It is a reminder of individual and organizational vulnerabilities and limitations in building community (McNerney, 1995). Organizations need time to develop the necessary depth of leadership to be able to learn from each other. The rewards for all must come from achieving milestones along the way. But there will also be accidents and mistakes. Most of the remainder of this book is devoted to decreasing the occurrence of serious accidents and mistakes, learning from experience, and increasing the likelihood that more of the properties of an ideal health care system can be achieved, community by community, throughout the country.

3

An Overview of the Study

Eleven organized delivery systems (ODSs) were examined over a one- to four-year-period. These systems were selected based on five criteria: (1) that they have at least four owned operating entities; (2) that some systems serve a single or contiguous market (that is, they are geographically concentrated) while others serve multiple dispersed markets (that is, they involve more than one region); (3) that the systems be well established, with a strong likelihood of ongoing viability; (4) that the systems have stable leadership willing and able to commit to a longitudinal study; and (5) that there be a reasonable geographic representation across the country. The AHA's Health System Section was used as the source for selection. From the 268 systems listed in this directory in 1990, 35 systems were selected that met the above five criteria. Upon further discussion among the study team and contacts with the field, this list was narrowed to approximately twenty systems who were then contacted by phone and letter and sent a research prospectus describing the study's purpose and objectives. From these interactions, agreements were reached with initially ten systems. One system (Health Midwest, based in Kansas City, Missouri) participated in only the first year of the study. The Sisters of Providence Health System and the UniHealth health system participated in three years of the study but not the fourth year. During the fourth year, Mercy

Health Services and Sentara Health System were added to the study. Seven systems participated in all four years of the study.

Health Systems Integration Study Participants

Baylor Health Care System (Dallas, Texas)

EHS Health Care (Oak Brook, Illinois—presently Advocate Health Care, resulting from a merger of EHS and Lutheran General HealthSystem in January 1995)

Fairview Hospital and Health Care Services (Minneapolis–St. Paul, Minnesota)

Franciscan Health System (Aston, Pennsylvania)

Henry Ford Health System (Detroit, Michigan)

Mercy Health Services (Farmington Hills, Michigan)

Sentara Health System (Norfolk, Virginia)

Sharp HealthCare (San Diego, California)

Sisters of Providence Health System (Seattle, Washington)

Sutter Health (Sacramento, California)

UniHealth (Burbank, California)

Using 1994 data, the systems ranged in total assets from $476.2 million to $2.0 billion; in total revenues from $514.0 million to $2.0 billion; in the number of acute care units from three to twenty-three; and in the number of primary care, single-specialty, and multispecialty practices from zero to thirty-six. All of the study systems are affiliated in some manner with physician groups, ranging from independent practice associations (IPAs) to full ownership of the physician group. In addition, by the end of the study all but one study system had at least partial ownership of an insurance product with enrolled lives ranging from 153,000 to 1.5 million (figures include both HMO and PPO products).

In regard to the stages of market maturity described in Chapter Two, one was in Stage 1, an unstructured "access" market; four were in Stage 2, a "loose cost" market; three were in Stage 3, a consolidated "advanced cost" market; and two were in Stage 4, a strict managed care "value" market. One system (Franciscan) had both an East and West region. The East region was characterized by a Stage 2 market and the West (headquartered in Tacoma, Washington) by a Stage 3 market. Two systems—Baylor and Henry Ford—had substantial medical school–affiliated teaching activities, and five of the systems—Franciscan West, Fairview, Mercy, Sisters of Providence, and Sutter—had substantial involvement in rural health care delivery. Brief "organizational biographies" of each system are highlighted in Resource A. The systems studied are primarily hospital- or physician-led models of organized delivery systems as opposed to independent physician group–led systems/networks or insurance company–led systems/networks. Further, they are primarily local regional systems, with the exception of Franciscan, Mercy, and Sisters of Providence, which are multistate regional systems.

It is important to note that the systems were not selected based on their degree of integration on any dimension. In fact, baseline comparison of the selected systems with forty-nine other systems participating in a national conference on integration revealed that conference participants averaged 4.33 on a scale of overall system integration (on a 1 to 7 scale, with 1 = low integration and 7 = high integration) versus 4.25 for the study systems and 4.06 on clinical integration versus 3.76 for the study systems. Additional comparisons of the selected systems with thirty-five systems belonging to American Health Care Systems (AmHS) (currently AmHS/Premiere/Sun Health) revealed that AmHS systems averaged 2.87 (on a 1 to 5 scale) on perceived medical staff integration versus 2.24 for the study participants and 2.88 versus 2.48 for perceived clinical integration. Both differences are statistically significant at $p \leq .05$.

Finally, each set of study system leaders (that is, CEO and Strategic Planner or equivalent person) was asked to complete an integration checklist developed by Coddington, Moore, and Fischer

(1994) in a study of ten other health systems and group practices. The checklist covers such characteristics as "physicians in leadership position," "primary care physicians economically integrated," "financial incentives aligned," and "real-time communication systems and a common data base exist," with weights assigned to various response categories, such as 8 points for "have interconnected information system and common data base for hospital, physicians, and health plan(s)." The summary score has a theoretical range from 0 (not at all integrated) to 100 (fully integrated on all dimensions). The study systems' average score was 53 with a range from 26 to 86, compared with an average of 70.7 and a range from 28 to 96 in the Coddington, Moore, and Fischer study (1994).

The above comparisons indicate that while the study systems were not randomly selected and do not reflect the universe of all systems in the country, they were not selected as outstanding a priori examples of integration. None of the selection criteria were correlated with degree of integration. Rather, the study systems recognized the growing importance of integration and were committed to learning more about the phenomenon.

Study Framework

Figure 3.1 depicts the study's overall conceptual framework. As shown, the "generator" of integrated delivery systems must come from the vision, culture, strategy, and leadership of governing boards, top management team executives, and physician leaders associated with the system. These elements are discussed further in Chapter Seven. They are the "inputs" for the development of both the functional integration and the physician-system integration blocks, defined in Chapter Two. As shown in Figure 3.1, clinical integration is primarily influenced by the degree of functional integration and physician-system integration. Functional integration and physician-system integration are seen as "causally prior" to clinical integration because we believe it is not possible to create

Figure 3.1. Framework for Examining an Organized Delivery Systems.

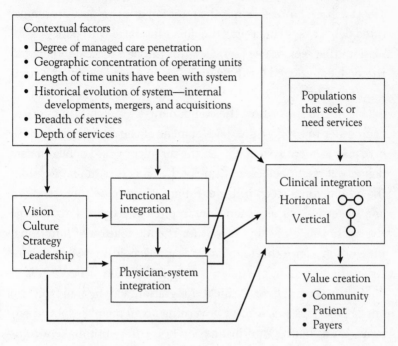

clinically integrated care without physicians who serve as the key decision makers in the process and without certain functions such as information systems and quality management in place. As defined in Chapter Two, clinical integration includes both horizontal and vertical integration. Of the two, vertical integration is more important because it represents the process by which the continuum of care is coordinated. In a strict sense, vertical integration refers to the direct ownership of different stages of the production process—for example, a system that owns all of its hospitals, primary care group practices, nursing homes, home health agencies, and so on. In this book, we will use the term *vertical integration* to also refer to *contractual* arrangements encompassing a variety of partnerships and strategic alliances among provider units (Kaluzny, Zuckerman, and Ricketts, 1995), as further discussed in Chapter Seven. Some have referred to these arrangements as "virtual integration" (Goldsmith, 1994). Clinical integration is the most important aspect of an organized delivery system, as it is the direct interface with patient populations that seek or need services. It is through clinical integration that value is created for the patient seeking services, for the community, and for payers.

Figure 3.2 shows how the components of integration build on each other to support the development of the community health care management system. Given the turbulent world of health care delivery, it might be best to think of the process as similar to building a home on a steep hillside. Pillars—vision, culture, strategy, and leadership of the system—are inserted into bedrock to become the anchoring and support rods for the foundation of functional integration. Once this foundation is in place, it is possible to construct the first floor, physician-system integration. Once this is in place, the second floor, clinical integration, can be built in. The entire process is overseen by governing board members of the system who recognize that just as one house does not make a community, one organized delivery system, particularly in a large metropolitan area, will not be able to support a community health care management system alone. Rather, as previously noted, linkages must be forged across the organized delivery systems within metropolitan markets to develop a community-wide health management system. Community-wide Health Information Networks (CHINS) may play a key role in the development of such systems.

A third way to view what is needed to create community health care management systems is to think about the value chain of health care delivery as shown in Figure 3.3. *Value* is defined as a *relationship* between quality attributes desired by consumers and the price they must pay to obtain those attributes. Thus, value in health care is created when, for a given price paid by consumers, a given organized delivery system provides more of the quality attributes desired by consumers than do competing systems. Alternatively, value is created when, for a given constellation of quality attributes

Figure 3.2. Building the House of Integration.

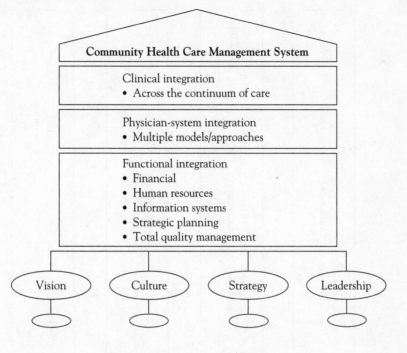

desired by consumers, a given organized delivery system provides them at a lower price than another. The term *value chain* is used in considering production processes in industry and manufacturing. All of the elements needed to produce a good or service are considered, and analysis is then conducted to determine at what points in the value chain the most value can be added. Consideration is given to those points in the chain that can be eliminated altogether and to those parts that might best be combined to add value.

In Figure 3.3, the first row depicts some of the different stakeholders that health care delivery systems must satisfy. It is important to note that each of these groups may "value" different outcomes and have different sets of expectations. This means that how value is created for individual patients, for example, may differ from how it is created for employers.

Figure 3.3. The Value Chain of Health Care Delivery.

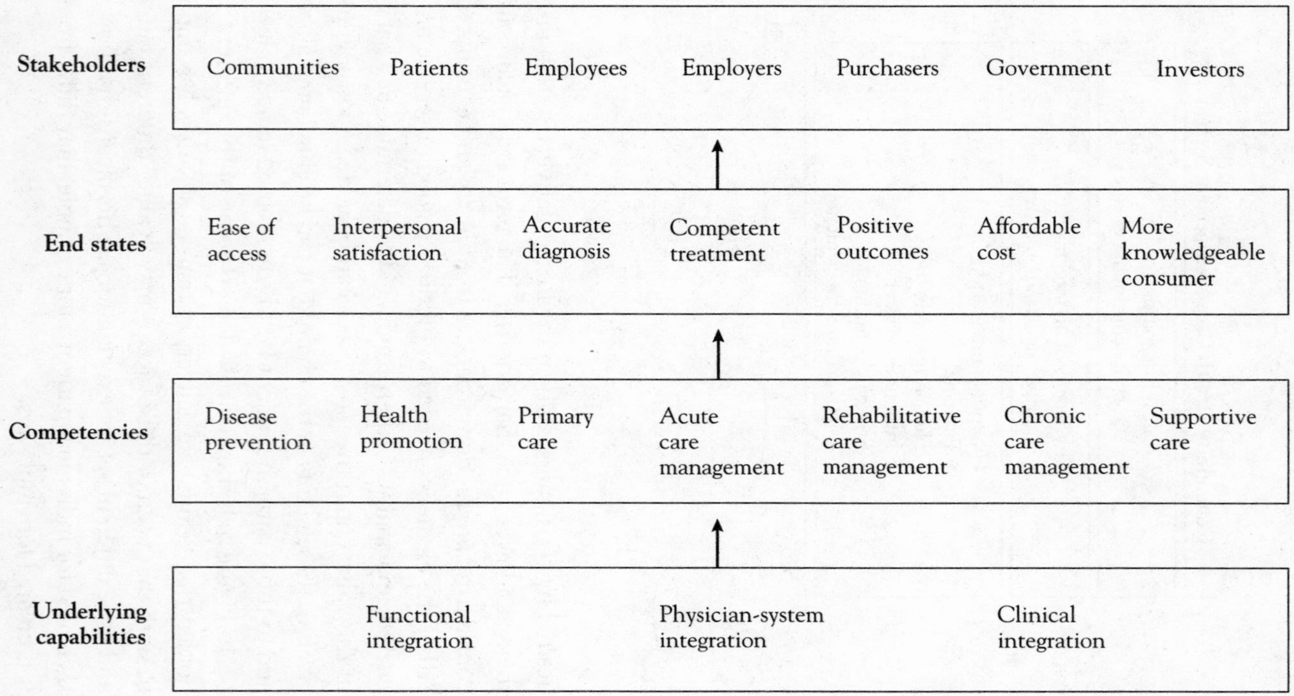

Stakeholders	Communities	Patients	Employees	Employers	Purchasers	Government	Investors

End states	Ease of access	Interpersonal satisfaction	Accurate diagnosis	Competent treatment	Positive outcomes	Affordable cost	More knowledgeable consumer

Competencies	Disease prevention	Health promotion	Primary care	Acute care management	Rehabilitative care management	Chronic care management	Supportive care

Underlying capabilities	Functional integration	Physician-system integration	Clinical integration

The second row depicts the desired end states, and the next row shows the processes that produce the end states. These processes are often thought of as constituting the *continuum of care* but can also be thought of as competencies that an organized delivery system must possess. *Competency* is defined as a specific product or service that an organization can deliver to a specific market or group of consumers (Prahalad and Hamel, 1990).

The fourth row depicts the underlying capabilities of an organized delivery system that enable it to leverage its competencies. A *capability* is best considered as a set of organizational skills and processes that leverage an entire value chain and are inherently cross-functional processes (Stalk, Evans, and Shulman, 1992). Underlying capabilities are usually more difficult to achieve than are competencies, and are therefore more difficult for competitors to imitate. Examples of underlying capabilities in organizations outside of health care include General Electric's ability to manage change, 3M's ability to innovate through creative use of organizational design, Motorola's capabilities in total quality management, and WalMart's logistical support system. In similar fashion, the potential underlying capabilities of health care delivery systems reside in their functional integration capacities (such as their information systems and total quality management processes), their ability to integrate physicians into systems of care, and their ability to achieve meaningful levels of clinical integration.

Why More Integration?

There is a trend for organizations in other industries to outsource functions, creating what some have called the "hollow" or "network" organization (Miles and Snow, 1986, 1994). The objective is to focus on the organization's core competency and then purchase the necessary inputs from others who specialize in those inputs or supportive processes. Why is health care apparently moving in the other direction? Why the rush to integration? We believe the answers lie in understanding the nature of health care and the new payment incentives.

The Nature of Health Care

It is important to recognize the *complex* and *interdependent* nature of health care. The human body is an enormously complex organism—entire industries spend and generate hundreds of millions of dollars to study and treat it. When a "breakdown" in the organism occurs, whether as minor as an upper respiratory infection or as major as pancreatic cancer, it generates multiple needs that are not easily isolated. Untreated, the respiratory infection can result in hospitalization and post-hospitalization care. The person with pancreatic cancer is likely to require a variety of caregivers in a variety of settings during the course of the illness. Breakdowns in health, as well as efforts to promote health, require the experience and expertise of many different kinds of people. This results in the almost inherent fragmentation of delivery we have noted previously. Specialized expertise needs to be coordinated to meet patients' treatment and health status objectives—in other words, the various components of the caregiving process need to become more integrated.

From an organizational perspective, it is helpful to consider the nature of interdependence. In his seminal work, *Organizations in Action*, Thompson (1967) defined three forms of interdependence—pooled, sequential, and reciprocal. In *pooled* interdependence, two or more activities of an organization do not need to be directly coordinated because they do not depend on each other for resources or inputs. The only coordination needed is at the level of the firm overall, where the outputs of the various activities must be pooled or brought together. An example is the retail clothing industry, in which organizations do not need to directly coordinate the efforts of those who make dresses and suits but rather must arrange to display them to potential buyers in an attractive and convenient manner. In *sequential* interdependence, one set of activities (Set B) depends on another set (Set A) in order to do its work, but A does not depend on B. Another set of activities (Set C) may in turn depend on B, but B does not depend on C. Sequential interdependence is typical of most assembly line work such as that traditionally associated with automobile manufacturing and food processing. *Reciprocal* interdependence is a more complex process in which A and B depend on each other for resources and inputs in order to do their work. They exchange resources in an ongoing reciprocal fashion in order to provide a good or service. Examples include producing movies or teaching a class. In movie production, the actors clearly need the producer and the cameras, and at the same time the producer and cameras need the actors, resulting in a dynamic interplay of several "takes" for important scenes, adjustment of lighting and camera angles, changes in settings and script, and changes in the actor's performance. Similarly, students depend on teachers to learn, but what teachers do greatly depends on student reaction and input. They influence each other in the process of learning and knowledge production. Reciprocal interdependence is a higher form of interdependence requiring more complex and fluid coordination and integration mechanisms. Health care delivery is characterized by a high degree of reciprocal interdependence, thus demanding a high degree of integration.

New Payment Incentives

The second reason for the increased interest in integration is that the new forms of payment—particularly capitated or lump-sum payment for a predetermined set of services to defined populations—provide financial incentives for more integrated delivery. Not only must organizations have enough services to cover the continuum of care but they must also reduce duplication of services, eliminate retesting, reduce missed appointments, and so on because all of these are costly. For providers to maintain their base of patients, the expectations of employees for an integrated, well-coordinated experience must be met.

At the same time, it is important to reiterate that organized delivery systems do not need to salary all physicians or own all components of the delivery process. Some can be outsourced or contracted out through a variety of partnerships and alliances. But the system must be able exert influence on the partnerships and alliances in order to ensure that integrated delivery occurs. The decision whether or not to own all components or contract for some of them depends on the organization's comparative expertise in the area of interest, the amount of capital available, the relative costs involved, the organization's culture, its history and traditions, its geographic location, its attitude toward risk, and the nature of competitive and collaborative forces in its market.

Because of the unique characteristics of health care we have just discussed, the central thesis of this book is that organized delivery systems that have higher levels of functional, physician-system, and clinical integration will better meet patient, payer, and community needs. They will be more successful in meeting their financial and related objectives. We must reiterate that we are talking about behavioral integration and not legal or "on paper" integration.

Working Hypotheses

To focus the study, a number of working hypotheses were developed in each area of interest.

Functional Integration

The primary components of functional integration are financial management, human resources, information systems, strategic planning, and continuous quality improvement/total quality management (hereafter referred to as CQI/TQM). As we have discussed (see also Figure 3.2), these represent the foundation upon which physician-system and clinical integration are built. Integration of these functional processes refers to the extent to which they serve all components of the system in a coordinated, cost-effective fash-

ion. Elsewhere, we have referred to these as exhibiting the properties of "systemness" (Shortell, Morrison, and Friedman, 1990).

An example of a high degree of functional integration would be
financial management practices and policies—regarding such issues
as budgeting, accounts receivable and cash management, and, in
particular, capital allocation across operating units—that are shared
and standardized among operating units. A high level of human
resources integration would be reflected, for example, in common
guidelines for wage and salary administration; employee orientation
and continuing education programs that emphasize the system as
opposed to individual operating units; cross-training of personnel;
and job posting across the system. A high level of systemness in
information systems would be reflected in the development of systems that link providers and patients across the system's continuum
of care. Relevant clinical and financial information would flow from
provider to provider and setting to setting with data available for
both internal continuous improvement of quality and for meeting
external accountability reporting requirements. Strategic planning
integration would mean that all units' plans are created within the
context of systemwide guidelines, assumptions, and strategic objectives. Finally, CQI/TQM would exhibit a high degree of systemness
when there is a systemwide plan for continuous improvement that
incorporates the entire continuum of care, where structures are in
place to diffuse the learning and best practices across the system,
and where system members receive common training and exposure
to CQI/TQM methodologies and principles.

As shown in Figure 3.1, we believe that a system's vision, culture, strategic orientation, and leadership will be positively associated with its degree of functional integration. In the current study,
we view vision and leadership as being primarily reflected in the
system's culture and strategic orientation. We hypothesize that systems with cultures that emphasize participation, mutual support,
risk taking, and innovation rather than rules, regulations, and hierarchy will be more functionally integrated. This is because rules,

regulations, and hierarchy get in the way of coordinating activities across units, whereas involvement, participation, mutual support, and willingness to try new approaches are more likely to be associated with cross-unit functional integration.

We also hypothesize that systems with *strategic orientations* that are more like those of prospectors and analyzers will be more functionally integrated than those with strategic orientations more like defenders and reactors. Briefly, a prospector strategy is characterized by the system's attempting to be the first to the market by being innovative and willing to try new services and new arrangements and by promoting risk taking (Miles and Snow, 1978). In contrast, an organization with a defender strategy attempts to defend its current main business or service line and simply tries to be more efficient in that domain. An analyzer strategy is somewhat more balanced between a defender and a prospector. An analyzer is not likely be first to market but will often follow the prospector with a more carefully developed product or service or will attempt to serve a niche segment that is unoccupied by the prospector. Organizations with prospector and analyzer strategic orientations need to move more quickly, necessitating coordinated action across units. Defenders focused on making existing units more efficient or reactors who do not have a coherent strategy are less likely to have functional support activities that are integrated. This is particularly likely to be true in the case of health systems in which hospital operating units have been the traditional core of business. To the extent that systems continue to emphasize acute inpatient care—a defender strategy—they are likely to emphasize functional support processes that focus on individual hospitals. This creates a barrier to developing processes that cut across the continuum of care.

Regarding the *contextual* factors shown in Figure 3.1, we expect that managed care penetration, geographic concentration of operating units, historical evolution of systems through more internal development rather than through mergers and acquisitions, and depth of services offered will each be positively associated with a greater degree of functional integration.

Managed care penetration creates incentives for systems to be-come more functionally integrated; geographic concentration and development of the system from within both make it easier to func-tionally integrate (mergers and acquisitions make it more difficult); and greater depth of services provides greater opportunities and potential economies of scale for functional integration.

In contrast, we expect the contextual factors involving the length of time that operating units have been with the system and the breadth of the system in terms of the number of different types of ser-vices offered will be *negatively* related to functional integration. It is important to recognize that although breadth and depth of services are considered "contextual" factors, they are not exogenous: they are influenced by the system culture, leadership, strategy, and vision.

The greater the length of time that units have been with a sys-tem, the greater the opportunity they have had to develop and rein-force their own functional support activities and autonomy, which serve as barriers to cross-unit integration efforts (Shortell, Gillies, and others, 1993). At the same time, systems with operating units that have belonged for longer periods of time are probably more likely to have evolved internally. As previously noted, we expect such systems to be more functionally integrated than systems that have been built through mergers and acquisitions, because they do not have the challenges of integrating newly emerged units. Thus, to the extent that the measures of length of time that operating units have been with a system and historical evolution through internal development are correlated, the predicted effects may cancel each other out. As for breadth of services, we expect that systems exhibiting a greater breadth of services will face more chal-lenges in functionally integrating such support processes as finan-cial management, human resources, information systems, strategic planning, and CQI/TQM.

Physician-System Integration

As shown in Figure 3.1, we believe physician-system integration will be influenced by the degree of functional integration of the key

processes discussed above, the system's culture and strategic orientation, and the contextual factors. The functional integration
processes serve as the foundation for building physician-system integration. Information systems and TQM processes are particularly
important because they directly affect physicians' ability to provide
more cost-effective coordinated care across the continuum.

Cultures that emphasize involvement, participation, mutual support, and a willingness to consider new approaches to physician
relationships (ranging from independent practice associations, to
physician-hospital organizations (PHOs), to salary and equity models) are hypothesized to be positively associated with greater physician-system integration than hierarchical, bureaucratic cultures that
emphasize rational efficiency objectives. Because most physicians
have traditionally been small businesspersons and are not used to
working in teams, let alone large organizations, they have a natural
aversion to rules and regulations that are perceived as standing in
the way of expressing their professional judgment and autonomy
(Freidson, 1970a, 1970b; Scott, 1982).

There is no straightforward prediction regarding the relationship between strategic orientation and physician-system integration
because we believe it depends significantly on the physicians
involved. For example, primary care physicians are likely to favor a
prospector strategic orientation because of the emphasis of this strategy on building new practice models that emphasize primary care
networks and that economically support primary care physicians.
Specialists, on the other hand, are more likely to be supportive of a
defender strategy that continues to emphasize acute inpatient care
and that still sees primary care efforts as primarily a way to fill hospital beds and increase referrals to specialists. It may be that an analyzer approach incorporating aspects of both the prospector and
defender might best promote physician-system integration.

Regarding contextual factors, we believe that managed care penetration will be positively associated with physician-system integration because it will create incentives for most physicians to align
with one system or another. Geographic concentration will be pos-

itively associated because it facilitates interaction among physicians and is also likely to be correlated with physician referral patterns. The length of time units have been with the system may have a positive association with physician-system integration to the extent that the units themselves (primarily the hospital in this case) are well integrated into the system. Where units are not well integrated, we expect less physician-system integration because physicians primarily identify with a system through their relationship with a hospital, although this is beginning to change as the primary relationship becomes that with a physician group or a PHO. We expect that systems that have evolved primarily internally (as opposed to those built more through mergers and acquisitions) will be positively associated with physician-system integration because of physician familiarity with the system. Greater system breadth of services will be negatively associated with physician integration because of the diversity of services offered, resulting in greater opportunities for conflict regarding how resources should be spent. Finally, system depth of services will be positively associated with physician-system integration because of the opportunities for physicians involved with similar services to work together—recognizing that other variables will influence whether or not this actually occurs.

Clinical Integration

As shown in Figure 3.1, clinical integration will be positively influenced by physician-system and functional integration, as well as culture, strategy, and the contextual factors. Because of the physician's central role in the delivery of medical and health services, we believe that the most important determinant of clinical integration is physician-system integration. A delivery system cannot achieve a high degree of clinical integration without having a substantial number of physicians who identify with the system, use it, and who are substantively involved in its management and governance. And, as we have discussed, physician-system integration is very much influenced by functional integration, culture, strategic orientation, and the contextual factors. We believe that these variables probably also exert an independent influence directly on clinical integration itself. Thus, all of the functional integration processes—information systems, quality management, and so on—are expected to be positively associated with clinical integration, as is a system culture that is more participative, involving, supportive, and innovation oriented.

As to strategic orientation, however, we believe that an *analyzer* strategy is most likely to support clinical integration efforts rather than a pure prospector or pure defender strategy. A prospector strategy will do a good job of assembling the pieces of the continuum of care but may not do as good a job integrating them. Prospectors often spread themselves thin pursuing new areas of opportunity without consolidating and implementing the new products or services that have materialized. In contrast, defenders will be slow to develop even the new products and services needed to provide clinical integration across the continuum of care. The analyzer, on the other hand, is more likely to pursue new possibilities with "deliberate speed," looking for market niches to fill in the continuum of care and integrating the pieces as they are acquired.

Finally, the contextual factors are expected to exert effects on clinical integration similar to those previously discussed in regard to functional integration and physician-system integration. Of particular importance will be the breadth of services (which makes it more difficult to clinically integrate) and depth of services (which makes it easier to clinically integrate) associated with a given system. Also, the greater the geographic concentration of the system's operating units, the greater the degree of clinical integration. We also expect that managed care penetration greatly increases a system's need to integrate services across the continuum.

Value Creation—Financial Performance

While ultimately one would wish to measure "value creation" for the community, patients, and payers, this was beyond the resources of the current study. For example, we would like to assess the impact of clinical integration and physician-system integration on the overall cost of care per episode of illness, on clinical outcomes of care, on functional health status, on patient satisfaction for specific conditions and, ultimately, on community health status and well-being. But this is an enormously daunting task in which the measurement tools themselves are still in the relatively early stages of development (Iezzoni, 1994; Ware, 1993). Further, study designs are needed that can isolate the impact of clinical and physician-system integration from multiple other factors that influence community health status and well-being such as education, income, safety, and environmental factors.

Given resource and data limitations, the only reliable comparative performance data available were selected measures of system and operating-unit financial performance. We hypothesize that systems that are more clinically integrated enjoy better financial performance as measured by such indicators as cash flow, total margin, and related variables we will discuss further below. This is because clinical integration results in more cost-effective patient care delivery that both attracts more revenue through acquiring more patients and enrolled lives and decreases costs by eliminating duplicate services and by reducing errors and rework. We also expect that physician-system integration may exert some independent direct effects on financial performance other than through its influence on clinical integration. We expect this to operate primarily through the greater revenue production potential of physicians organized into groups that are positioned to take on risk and win managed care contracts.

Methods and Measures

The study involved extensive collection of both primary and secondary data over a period of four years, complemented by two summers of field work involving on-site interviews with system participants. Resource B lists the various data collection instruments and activities, the type of data collected, when the data were collected, and what the data measured. Many of the actual measures used are discussed in Gillies and others (1993) and Devers and others (1994). In addition, as noted in Resource B, more detail on these measures is available from the authors.

In the following chapters, descriptive data on functional, physician-system, and clinical integration are reported along with the most salient findings. Because the potential number of cases at the system level is only between nine and twelve systems/regions, examination of the relationships is limited to bivariate Spearman rank correlation. Only correlations that are significant at the .05 level are discussed, and most correlations generally ranged from 0.50 to 0.90 in magnitude. Relevant findings from multiple regression analyses carried out at the operating unit are also noted.

4

Functional Integration

Coordinating the System's Components

Human resources, outcomes management, central-
ized budgeting and information are core integrating
mechanisms, and without them you cannot achieve
integration to manage the life of a patient over time.
John Lee, *regional vice president,*
Sisters of Providence, in Cerne, 1994, p. 39.

We have defined functional integration as the extent to which key support functions and activities (such as financial management, human resources, strategic planning, information management, marketing, and quality improvement) are coordinated *across operating units* so as to add the greatest overall value to the system. In the most general sense, integration involves shared or common policies and practices for each of these functions. However, integration does not mean mere centralization and/or standardization; that is, centralization and standardization do not automatically translate into a high level of integration. The degree of integration depends on what the consequences of centralization/standardization are.

The key to functional integration is that the functional processes serve all the components of the system in a coordinated manner. The good of the system is paramount. The purpose behind the integration of human resource functions, for example, is not merely the establishment of common policies and processes but rather the establishment of those *that facilitate movement of resources within and between operating units to where they are needed at any particular time*. The more the human resource functions of a system allow the system to use its human resources to its best advantage, the more functionally integrated the human resources policies and processes are. Financial management processes are more integrated the more they allow budgeting and capital allocation that emphasize the needs of the system overall instead of individual operating-unit goals. Integrated financial management functions enable the system to shift resources around the system so as to maximize the system's capacity. The more the strategic plans of the various units in the system are based on a set of common guidelines and goals that are designed to enhance the *system*, the higher the degree of integration. Integration of information systems occurs when there is an exchange of data within and among a system's operating units that promotes cost-effective care across the continuum and overall clinical and fiscal responsibility. Quality improvement efforts are more integrated the more they are common or shared throughout the system and promote the mutual learning required for the continuous improvement of quality.

Not all functions of a system, however, must necessarily be integrated to the same extent. Depending on the design of the system, some functions may be more important to integrate than others. As Williams notes:

> Centralize and standardize only where appropriate. Successful healthcare management companies appear to be decentralizing many functions directly related to patient care delivery and beginning to restructure the way patient care is delivered. . . . At the same time, they are continuing to centralize, standardize, and/or consolidate those staff functions where there are significant economies of scale and/or expertise to be gained. [1992, pp. 39–40]

Williams indicates CQI/TQM, planning, budgeting, information, and communication as being especially critical.

Primary Findings

The measures of functional integration developed in the study are based on perception, collected at multiple time points using self-administered structured (closed-ended) questionnaires. Based on management responses obtained from these questionnaires, measures were computed for nine functional areas as well as for overall functional integration. Table 4.1 presents the study means, standard deviations, and ranges for the perceived functional integration measures for individual functional areas and the overall functional integration measure.

Most of the functional integration measures were collected at two time points, 1991 and 1992, but two of the measures, information services and quality assurance, were collected at three time points, 1991, 1992, and 1994. Since perceived overall functional integration is based on the complete set of functional areas, overall functional integration is available only for 1991 and 1992.

Degree of Integration

A number of observations can be made regarding the measures of perceived functional integration. While study participants have achieved a moderate level of functional integration in some areas, the challenges of integration remain for a number of others. For the most part, the mean values for integration of the various functions hover around 3.0, the midpoint of the scale. Perceptions of integration are highest (3.4) for financial management operating policies. Two functions, support services and information services, have the lowest values (both with 2.4 in 1991 and 2.5 in 1992). The continued low value of information systems is especially noteworthy given the importance of information systems for physician-system and clinical integration.

Table 4.1. Measures of Perceived Functional Integration.

Concept or measure	Fiscal year 1991 $\overline{x}$ (Standard deviation; Range)	Fiscal year 1992 $\overline{x}$ (Standard deviation; Range)	Fiscal year 1994 $\overline{x}$ (Standard deviation; Range)
Human resources	2.9 (.45; 2.3–3.6)	3.0 (.31; 2.3–3.3)	
Support services	2.4 (.39; 2.0–3.3)	2.5 (.41; 2.0–3.4)	
Culture	3.2 (.43; 2.3–3.7)	3.2 (.44; 2.3–3.7)	
Strategic planning	3.1 (.36; 2.5–3.5)	3.1 (.35; 2.4–3.6)	
Quality assurance	3.0 (.40; 2.6–3.9)	3.0 (.27; 2.5–3.3)	2.9 (.31; 2.5–3.5)
Marketing	2.8 (.50; 2.2–3.7)	2.7 (.28; 2.2–3.1)	
Information services	2.4 (.31; 2.0–2.8)	2.5 (.25; 2.1–2.9)	2.3 (.24; 2.0–2.7)
Financial management–resource allocation	3.0 (.45; 2.4–3.8)	3.2 (.32; 2.5–3.6)	
Financial management–operating policies	3.4 (.27; 2.9–3.9)	3.4 (.24; 3.0–3.9)	
Overall functional integration	3.0 (.28; 2.5–3.4)	3.0 (.20; 2.6–3.2)	

Note: $\overline{x}$ = mean

In addition, little, if any, improvement (at least in terms of the mean values of the perceptions) is indicated from 1991 to 1992, or even to 1994 for the two functions for which 1994 data are available. As shown in the table, the study systems have not seen any increase in functional integration, although there have been some individual system changes (as can be seen from the minimum and maximum values). However, this may be as much due to changes in perceptions of what needs to be done as to lack of actual changes in integration.

In related analyses, corporate managerial respondents generally reported higher values than did the operating-unit managerial respondents—significantly higher on culture, strategic planning, marketing, financial planning–resources allocation, and financial planning–operating policies, but significantly lower on support services (Gillies and others, 1993). In fact, additional analysis shows that in general, physicians have an even more positive assessment of integration than corporate management has, and board respondents have the most positive assessment. The differences between corporate and noncorporate respondents may be attributed to several reasons. First, the noncorporate operating-unit management respondents are on the front line, so to speak, actually trying to implement the integration policies. As a result, issues and problems of the integration process may be more evident to them, and thus they see less integration than do corporate respondents. System-level respondents, on the other hand, view the process from an overall system perspective, and thus see more integration. In addition, each group of individuals may see what they want to see—operating-unit management views integration as a threat and denies its presence, whereas system management desires more integration and sees more integration than there actually is.

Other Key Relationships

In addition to the descriptive analysis of perceived overall functional integration and its components, the relationships between functional integration (focusing only on the overall functional integration measure) and other factors were examined. These analyses show only a few variables that were significantly associated with perceived overall functional integration:

- The greater the number of hospitals in a system, the higher the perceived level of overall functional integration. This likely reflects economies of scale.

- Systems with higher perceived cultural integration were also likely to have higher perceived overall functional integration.

Contrary to the hypotheses proposed in Chapter Three, no relationship was found at the system level between perceived overall functional integration and group culture, strategic orientation, managed care penetration, internal development of the system, breadth of services, depth of services, or average length of time that the operating units have been with the system.

Standardization

Another approach to examining functional integration is to assess the extent to which functions are standardized across operating units; that is, the extent to which all operating units within a system use the same approaches, policies, practices, and guidelines in carrying out functions and activities. Standardization of functions was evaluated using a questionnaire containing forty-nine yes/no questions related to selected functional support areas (listed below). This was completed by each of the study system's strategic planners. For each functional area the degree of standardization was determined by computing the percentage of yes responses, with 0 percent meaning that none of the items was standardized and 100 percent meaning that all items were standardized throughout the system. Although this approach does not fully incorporate the notion that standardization (as indicated by the same approach, policies, practices, and guidelines) actually facilitates the coordination of services and adds value to the system, the findings are consistent with the perceptual data presented in Table 4.1; namely, information systems integration was perceived as among the least integrated areas and financial management operating policies were the most highly integrated. In increasing order of standardization, the functional areas examined and the degree of standardization as a percentage are as follows: information services, 22 percent; quality assurance/improvement, 26 percent; human resources, 32 percent; culture, 33 percent; other (including managed care contracting, administrative practices, and new product and service development), 43 percent; support services, 50 percent; strategic planning, 55 percent; and financial management, 72 percent. The average percentage of items indicated as standardized over the eight functional areas is 42 percent (Devers and others, 1994, p. 10). As noted above, these standardization measures do not necessarily incorporate the notion of added value that is implied by integration. In fact, the perceived integration measure is significantly correlated (using Spearman rank correlation) with its corresponding standardization measure only for the functional areas of human resources, financial management, and quality assurance. Integration and standardization are not correlated for support services, strategic planning, culture, and information systems. Generally, the standardization measures are not significantly related to the contextual and background measures used in the study.

Summary of the Primary Findings

Overall there is little consistent statistical support for the relationships between the factors hypothesized to be associated with functional integration and functional integration itself. It may be that our hypotheses are not valid; in other words, perhaps the factors suggested do not influence functional integration. An alternative explanation is that the perceived functional integration measures may not be valid measures of real functional integration, especially in terms of assessing the degree to which integration adds value to the system. It may be necessary to develop additional objective measures other than standardization. However, it may also be that participating systems are still in the relatively early stages of the integration process and thus the patterns are not yet clearly established or observable. This may be particularly true in such areas as information systems and TQM.

Barriers and Challenges

Many health care systems are attempting to promote functional integration. However, based on our examination they will confront a number of barriers in their attempts to achieve integration. These obstacles include the following: (1) lack of understanding of integration, (2) inability to identify the key functions to integrate, (3) lack of operating-unit commitment to the integration strategy, (4) continued focus on the operating unit, especially the hospital, (5) lack of geographic concentration of operating units, (6) lack of trained personnel, and (7) inadequate information systems.

Lack of Understanding

In many systems there is a lack of understanding as to what integration means—whether it be system, functional, physician-system, or clinical. Operating-unit personnel often perceive system attempts at integration as merely an attempt by the corporate people to usurp power. System leaders have not provided a design of the organized health care system nor a rationale for its development. Given the constant change in the health care environment, there is perhaps no model of the end-state system but rather a series of constantly evolving models that change as the structure of health care changes. However, in many systems only a privileged few have a vision of at least the basic outlines and goals of an organized delivery system, and only they may understand that a functionally integrated system should be better able to adapt itself to future conditions.

Inability to Identify Key Functions to Integrate

Another major problem is not knowing which functions will better serve the system if standardized or centralized and which are more beneficial if not; which functions are appropriately the responsibility of the operating units and which should be done at the regional or system levels. Should marketing be a standardized function? Human resources? Financial management? In part the answer to these questions is dependent on external factors such as market environment. However, part of the inability to determine which processes need to be integrated comes from a basic lack of understanding as to what the core business of a modern health care system is. The new core business has shifted from acute inpatient care to primary care, wellness, and the continuum of care. The need to integrate functions must be judged on the basis of the impact of such an action on the creation of a seamless continuum of care and what is best for the patient. (Cerne, 1994).

Lack of Operating-Unit Commitment to Integration

Another major barrier is the unwillingness of some of the system's operating units—especially those that in the past were, and may continue to be, the system's main cash source—to join in the system's integration efforts. For example, many systems are unable to convince the "cash cow" (that is, the operating unit that is the major source of revenue for a system) to accept the system strategy. The system may allow the cash cow to proceed with its own plans as long as it has the ability to fund them. Or the cash cow may be allowed to lead the entire system in a direction that benefits itself more than the system overall. The more successful units often do not want to integrate financial functions because they do not want to give up control of revenues and share their bounty with other components of the system. In addition, in a number of systems many of the operating units are reluctant to financially support system integration activities. There are other cases where some system operating units have balked, often out of feelings of superiority, at joining such functions as human resources with other system operating units. In general, there is often little willingness to sacrifice individual operating units for the good of the system or to see how helping others in the system actually benefits all of the system's components.

Continued Focus on the Hospital

Integration is also inhibited by the inability of the systems to overcome the hospital paradigm, from both the system's and the individual's perspectives. Hospitals remain the focus for many systems. Some of the systems continue to base their growth strategies on acquiring or affiliating with other hospitals, often to extend the system's geographical coverage, rather than basing growth on acquiring or affiliating with other types of units along the continuum of care, such as physician groups and home care. It is questionable whether affiliations of these like types of units help the coordination of functions for the system as a whole as much as would the affiliation with more diverse units.

At the individual level, the hospital (or more generally, operating unit) focus means that many of the individuals in the system continue to identify with and owe their allegiances to the individual operating unit. As a result, efforts to integrate various functions are hindered because operating unit–oriented employees consider the needs of the system as secondary to those of the hospital. For example, integrated human resource policies may require employees with enough flexibility to work at whichever system site has needs at a particular time; operating unit–oriented people may not be able or willing to do this.

Lack of Geographic Concentration of Operating Units

A barrier related to the problem of overemphasis on hospitals is the geographic spread of the hospitals and other operating units. As mentioned above, in the past (and, in some cases, even in the present), many systems viewed development as acquiring more hospitals and extending their geographic coverage. Little forethought was given to coordination of the various operating units and pro-

vision of the full continuum of care. As a result, a mapping of system facilities often shows a set of disjointed operating units for
which there may be little hope of coordinating services. The lack
of geographic concentration of the hospital units often reduces the
likelihood of integration. Again using the human resource function as an example, the benefits of common human resource policies and guidelines may not be realized if the various operating
units are too far apart to allow personnel to be shifted from site to
site as the need arises.

Lack of Trained Personnel

Problems with personnel shifts relate not only to shifts from site to
site but also to shifts from function to function. Care for the patient
across the continuum requires a vast array of expertise in a number
of settings. Advances in technology have changed the requirements
of many jobs in the health care system. In addition, continuity of
care argues for patient contact with *fewer* people who have *more*
skills. However, a number of factors prevent systems from utilizing
system personnel to either the system's or the patient's best advantage. Most systems confront state and federal limitations (such as
licensing requirements and regulations) on the use of their personnel. Some systems also face union limitations. Even if these factors
are overcome, in many cases personnel with the necessary skills
(either specialized skills or multiple skills) are not available. Both
at the managerial and the clinical levels, systems are often trying to
perform "new (health care) world" tasks using personnel in "old
(health care) world" positions with "old world" skills. Efforts to integrate the human resource function or the support services function
are often thwarted.

Inadequate Information Systems

Another barrier to the development of functional integration concerns information systems. Underdeveloped information systems
inhibit physician-system and clinical integration; the lack of agreement about what the information system should be like inhibits

functional integration. Most of the study systems would characterize their information systems as woefully inadequate for their integration efforts. None of the participating systems has an information
system that can link all the key actors (for example, primary care
physician, hospital, home care) involved in the typical episode of
care for a patient or allow the system to effectively determine costs
and outcomes of treatments. Most systems do not even have a common patient identifier that would allow such information to be
linked between sites.

A few systems are relatively far along in assembling the pieces
of an information system, but none has implemented a full-scale system. There is no agreement as to what the components of such a
system should be, what information must be shared, and what does
not have to be shared. Many operating units have their own financial information system that some are reluctant to trade for either
a common system or at least one that allows for some compatibility with other operating units. Most operating units do have a clinical information system, limited as it may be, but are reluctant to
adopt systemwide standards that would allow cross-unit comparisons
and exchange of data as well as the merging of financial data with
clinical data to enable cost-effectiveness and cost-benefit analyses.

Key Success Factors and Some Best Practices

In spite of the barriers to integration, a number of the systems have
been able to increase not only the level of integration of specific
functions but also overall integration. These systems have used a
variety of mechanisms and approaches, no single one of which
would be adequate and not all of which would be suitable in all situations. However, a number of key success factors for functional
integration specifically and integration overall can be identified.

Strategic Plan

Key to integration is the development of a strategic plan that details
both a system's vision and goals and how the system intends to

achieve them. Ideally, the plan should be based on a population/ community-based health status needs assessment. It should be region-based and have physicians as the starting point. The strategic plan should also link short-run issues to long-run goals, the little picture to the big picture. An ODS must act in terms of its strategic plans and long-range goals, with the caveat that these plans and goals must be flexible enough to change with the changing needs of the population. For example, acquisition, merger, and affiliation efforts must be evaluated much more strategically in order to increase the likelihood that the system has the right pieces in the right places. Growth for growth's sake is no longer acceptable; greater attention must be given to population-based strategic planning emphasizing primary care and wellness rather than to acute care–based hospital planning. A successful ODS will evaluate all opportunities in relation to its population-based strategic plans and long-range goals: is this acquisition, merger, affiliation necessary to meet the needs of the population it serves? Does this move enhance system integration efforts? In addition, system leaders need to ensure that the system is strategically aligned: are management control systems matched with market strategy? Are incentives aligned with strategy? Are resources aligned with strategy? Proposed new services should be evaluated in terms of the system strategy.

Most of the systems in the study are paying increased attention to alignment of strategy and actions. Franciscan Health Systems has instituted systemwide technology assessment to help ensure that decisions are made in line with strategy. Henry Ford and Fairview increasingly incorporate population-based planning and community health status needs in their decision-making processes. And some of these systems have had opportunities to merge or affiliate with other systems or hospitals but declined to do so because the opportunities did not fit with their strategic plans. Alternatively, EHS Health Care determined that merging with Lutheran General HealthSystem was compatible with its strategic vision and joined with Lutheran to become Advocate Health Care in January 1995.

Leadership

Strong system leadership committed to the integration process is instrumental. System leaders must communicate the vision, strategy, and understanding of system integration throughout the system. Members of a system need to understand in real-world terms "system integration" and its component parts—functional, physician-system, and clinical integration. Increased understanding of integration should reduce fears and beliefs that integration, any integration, must surely adversely affect not only the individual (as with downsizing) but also the operating unit with which the individual identifies. Leaders need to emphasize the positive outcomes for the patient, the employee, the operating unit, and the system. Although system leaders may not be able to lay out a visual model of the end state, they must be able to explain the rationale behind the evolution of the system and present the model of the next stage.

The system leaders at each of the various study systems have made and continue to make concerted efforts to communicate to employees, boards, and affiliated personnel information concerning system culture, system goals, and the integration effort. Many use newsletters, retreats, and meetings as communication vehicles. The leaders at UniHealth also spread the message at systemwide ceremonies and events. At Henry Ford, the system CEO mails a special newsletter to trustees every two weeks detailing plans and developments.

Operating-Unit "Buy-In"

Gaining the operating units' "buy-in" of integration plans is crucial for success, and key to this is bringing the operating-unit leaders on board. Much attention must be given to these managers and associated implementation issues because these operating-unit leaders often do not see a need to change as quickly as system executives want. As a result they can derail any integration efforts.

There are a number of approaches to achieving operating-unit buy-in or at least reducing the insular orientation of a system's operating units. First, clear communication of the strategic role each operating unit is to play in the overall system/regional strategy can help alleviate operating-unit concerns. In addition, the system needs to find ways to change the focus of the operating-unit leaders from their own hospital to the system as a whole. Advocate Health Care and Fairview gave their hospital leaders cross-system management responsibilities. Sharp HealthCare and Franciscan Health Care West each consolidated hospital management into one team. The system can put chairs of the individual hospital boards on the overall system board and can create an office of governance for supporting all operating-entity and systemwide governance activities. Sentara has consolidated its governance boards into one. Many of these approaches are described further in Chapter Seven.

Culture

A strong system culture is important to the integration process. To become more functionally integrated, the system must develop ways to get beyond the unit-based orientation of many of those working within the system. This is not to say that individual unit variation cannot be allowed within the system. However, the overarching values should be those of the system, and primary allegiance should be to the system. Systems need to develop a strong culture (at least in terms of the core values) that will promote a system perspective and provide a platform for additional integration work. Williams views "management culture [as] one of the most powerful tools to promote integration" (1992, pp. 43–44). Although recognizing that changing a system's culture is difficult and time consuming, Williams suggests that system leaders should "assess and monitor your culture . . . [and] . . . focus culture changes on the areas that will truly further integration" (p. 44), which include decision making, organizational integration, management style, management compensation, and management development.

Cultural values can be enhanced by a number of means. Franciscan begins all board meetings with a discussion of the system's cultural values. Linking performance appraisal and compensation incentives to expression of the system's cultural values and to managerial behavior consistent with those values has helped promote the development of both Franciscan's and UniHealth's cultures. Some systems use special ceremonies and celebrations to reinforce system values and culture—for example, UniHealth's quarterly TEAM (Together Everyone Achieves More) rallies. Fairview uses "value clarification" processes by which the system values are communicated throughout the system. UniHealth has developed employee orientation videos that emphasize its culture. Henry Ford uses a systemwide newsletter to communicate its culture. As mentioned above, Henry Ford also mails a special trustees' newsletter to keep communication and system values visible.

A number of other mechanisms can be effective in developing a system orientation. For example, the use of cross-unit task forces can help facilitate joint programmatic efforts and get the members of a system more comfortable working with each other. Systems can institute joint programmatic planning and technology assessment planning across operating units. Cross-unit quality improvement activities are also used to help integrate various functional activities.

Systems should explore all opportunities to integrate, including initiating or expanding shared or common dietary, maintenance, housekeeping, security, and other support systems systemwide. Among the study systems, Sharp HealthCare, Sutter Health, and UniHealth have developed cross-unit support services. In addition, system councils, meetings, or task forces that cut across all operating entities in functional areas such as nursing, human resources, marketing, and planning can be established to encourage input on a systemwide basis. Advocate Health Care, Fairview, Henry Ford, and Sharp are among the study systems that have employed such systemwide groups.

CQI/TQM

Quality improvement activities, especially those utilizing CQI/TQM approaches, can be beneficial for integration efforts for several reasons. First, CQI/TQM is itself a management philosophy and approach that, if adopted by a system, helps define a common view of the world and thus a common culture. Secondly, the techniques of CQI/TQM tend to promote "systems" thinking by focusing on the linkages of processes and activities across functions and units. Finally, CQI/TQM projects often require personnel in different units or functional areas to work together. However, these CQI/TQM activities must be linked explicitly to the system's strategic priorities so that they add to the integration process of the system.

Most of the study systems use CQI/TQM as a means to strengthen cultural values and develop an overall sense of systemness. For example, Advocate, Fairview, Henry Ford, Mercy, Sentara, and Sharp all use cross-unit meetings, councils, teams, or task forces in their CQI/TQM efforts, thus building bridges among their various operating units and groups. Advocate and Sutter use the CQI process to build system identity in the lower levels of their system by involving co-workers in the selection of recipients of awards. Advocate, Henry Ford, and UniHealth use "system universities" that teach CQI methods to also promote the values and culture of the system.

Information Systems

An integrated information system is both a key factor in the development of an ODS and a consequence of that development: improving information systems helps system integration, and system integration helps develop information systems. Continued emphasis should be placed on developing clinical and management information systems as a foundation for facilitating overall integration efforts. However, information system development must be linked to the system's vision and strategic plan. The information needs of the various customers (community, patients, caregivers, payers, external accountability groups) must be defined. The information system(s) of an ODS should be designed around these needs and incorporate relational data that can link patients and providers across the continuum. Information system integration efforts should focus on information that can be used for "real-time" continuous improvement.

Although information system deficiencies should not be used as an excuse to avoid integration initiatives, information systems are nonetheless a key factor in achieving integration objectives. Recognizing this, many of the study's systems as well as other systems throughout the country are investing heavily in their information systems. The systems in the study are estimated to have invested between $30 million and $150 million over the course of the study. Group Health Cooperative of Puget Sound, a Seattle-based staff-model HMO with over 535,000 enrollees, has dramatically shifted its focus of capital investment from facilities to information systems. Over the next five years, Group Health Cooperative plans to invest over $100 million.

Systemwide Incentives for Individuals

Individual performance appraisal systems that emphasize cooperative interdependent work can be used to promote cross-system integration. Compensation and incentives should be aligned to reinforce cross-system and/or cross-functional integration achievements; performance appraisal and compensation incentives should be linked to expression of the system's cultural values and systemwide strategies, and to managerial behavior consistent with those values and strategies. Study systems are now typically basing about 50 to 60 percent of incentive pay for system executives on system performance levels and the remainder on individual unit operating performance and personal development goals and objectives.

Key to the success of these types of programs is a systematic human resource planning process that is linked to the system's strategic plan and identifies the needs and goals of the system (Williams, 1992). Training and development processes should foster integration by educating those involved to the desirability, concepts, and methodologies of integration. Human resource practices that build strong teams, reward team achievements on an ongoing basis, and provide for management continuity promote overall integration. Investment in cross-training employees and caregivers at all levels should be expanded. Also, systems should work to eliminate restrictive state and federal personnel licensing requirements and regulations. (We discuss this issue further in Chapter Eight.)

Performance Assessment of the System

Integration is not easily assessed, but it is important to have a means of monitoring a system's progress in becoming integrated. In order to evaluate progress in the integration effort, systems could develop an "integration scorecard" that would be shared throughout the system (Devers and others, 1994). Such a scorecard would track progress on specified measures over time. The measures would be linked to specific objectives and assigned to specific people and groups for purposes of accountability. Fairview has developed a set of systemwide critical success factors, goals, and milestones that aid in assessment. Henry Ford has several initiatives in this direction. It is developing a comprehensive system performance profile that can be used to meaningfully measure performance in four main areas: customer service, low-cost provider, system integration, and growth. In addition, Henry Ford's Consortium Research on Indicators of System Performance (CRISP) project is in the process of developing a more appropriate and comprehensive measurement approach for organized delivery systems that will give a "balanced scorecard" of system performance. These approaches are discussed further in Chapter Six.

Baylor Health Care System

When the Health Systems Integration Study began, the Dallas/Fort Worth marketplace in which Baylor Health Care System (BHCS) is located was characterized by few of the outside forces that motivate radical change in health care providers. Relative to other markets around the country, the Dallas market was highly utilized, with little managed care activity and relatively little concern about cost containment. As a result, BHCS was not very integrated. Instead, Baylor was a system with one major hospital, Baylor University Medical Center (BUMC), and a set of smaller community hospitals. These community hospitals seemed to be valued more for their ability to provide patients to BUMC than for their role in providing care for the community. However, Baylor leaders were concerned with the patterns they saw in other parts of the country and believed that these patterns would soon emerge in their area; the capitated world with its falling utilization rates was sure to affect their market at some point relatively soon. Although Baylor Health Care System had been extremely successful, it would need to be ready for this eventuality and not merely deal with it as it came. System leaders decided that transforming BHCS into a fully integrated health care delivery system would best position the system for this new world.

Obstacles to Integration

A number of barriers confronted BHCS as it began its integration journey. First, Baylor's past success made it difficult to motivate many members of the system to change or even to see the need for change. There was not enough pain to cause many of those in the system to question BHCS's traditional approach to health care delivery. Given the fact that many working for Baylor had been associated with the system (hospital) for a long period of time, there was great reluctance to remove or transfer those who would not or could not make any changes.

Another obstacle was the system's hospital focus. BHCS was based on acute inpatient care and traditional hospital CEO roles. Operating-unit boards had policy-making power. Different hospitals had different arrangements in terms of decision making and resources. Each operating unit was proud of its unique approach to caring for patients, which translated into a real unwillingness for each to adopt the other's methodology. Information systems were specific to operating units and very limited in scope; even within an operating unit, the information systems often could not talk to each other. The impact of this hospital focus was intensified by the system's concentration on Baylor University Medical Center. Baylor's evolution as a system can be seen as a series of smaller hospitals merging with Baylor University Medical Center. The attitude of many at BUMC appeared to be that its care and personnel were superior to other operating units in the system and that the other hospitals primarily functioned as feeders for BUMC. In certain respects, Baylor was more a confederation of hospitals than a system, and the differing perspectives of the operating units limited integration.

Culture presented another obstacle for BHCS. Baylor lacked a consistent culture throughout the system. Although religious values seem to be consistently shared across the system, there was no agreement on the core health system values. In addition, Baylor's CQI/TQM efforts and successes were not widely disseminated throughout the system and thus could not be used to develop a consistent culture. Most of the CQI/TQM work focused on BUMC, with very little conducted cross-system.

Another barrier to integration at Baylor was the lack of a consistent, focused strategic vision throughout the organization. Baylor did not have a formal strategic planning process. Operating-unit management did not really understand BHCS's overall system strategy. And the roles of each piece of Baylor's business—for example, BUMC and the community and specialty hospitals—were not articulated. Baylor did not have a clear view of what the system would look like in the future. Would BUMC be the hub of a hub-and-spoke system, or would each Baylor operating unit deliver a common set of predetermined services? What role would the hospitals play in the future? These fundamental questions did not have answers.

Progress Toward Functional Integration

In spite of all these obstacles, BHCS system leadership remained committed to the development of an organized delivery system. However, as they began to make integration plans, system leaders realized that they faced one more major stumbling block. Before they could even plan what they needed to do to become an ODS, BHCS needed to develop a clear idea of where the system needed to be. What does it mean for Baylor Health Care System to be a fully integrated health care delivery system? What are its core processes? How does the system know what to integrate functionally if it does not know what its core processes are? How does the system know what should be linked by its information system unless it understands its core processes?

In 1994, Baylor set out to determine its core processes and re-engineer around these processes. The *system as a whole* was the focus of this effort, not just BUMC or the various individual component operating units. Baylor created the System Integration Action Team, headed by the BHCS senior executive vice president and chief operating officer and consisting of twenty-eight Baylor employees and physicians. For fourteen months this team analyzed what kinds of work a Baylor integrated health care delivery system would need to perform to compete successfully in the changing health care market. The team defined the ultimate "customer" of the system to be the patient/member and named seven core processes:

1. Managing illness—focusing on the patient and caring for the patient after injury or onset of illness

2. Optimizing health and wellness—keeping people healthy

3. Coordinating member education and access to care—managing initial and ongoing contact with the member or potential patient

4. Developing, updating, and communicating BHCS strategies—keeping the other six core processes informed of the mission and priorities of BHCS and its plans for addressing the requirements of the marketplace

5. Capturing market—developing strategies to understand the requirements of the marketplace (patients and payers) and creating products and services to capture their business

6. Accessing and managing risk—requiring Baylor to develop risk products, that is, health plans in which Baylor becomes a part-

ner with managed care companies and physicians and assumes a financial risk in keeping enrollees healthy

7. Managing resources to support core processes—managing the services (for example, information systems, human resources, financial services, material services) that support the daily work of BHCS

The belief was that if Baylor could effectively arrange service delivery around these "value-added" processes, the consequences would be improvements in service quality, reductions in waste and rework, improvements in cycle time, and reductions in operating costs. Above all, the health care system would keep a defined population healthy.

Having defined the core processes, the Baylor team embarked on a multiyear project that would reengineer the system into a fully integrated health system. Beginning with "developing, updating, and communicating strategies," teams have been or will be launched for each of the core processes. In addition, subprocess teams in areas such as medication administration, elective surgery, and procurement have also been launched. BHCS has set a target date of January 1, 1997 for achieving initial integration objectives.

Keys to Success at Baylor

If Baylor continues to be successful in the future, the reason in part lies with forward-thinking leadership that was interested in integration before the marketplace dictated it. Although early efforts may not have been spectacular, BHCS leaders have been persistent in their efforts to integrate their system. They have been willing to reexamine their plans and actions and to change their approach as needed.

Lessons from the Baylor Experience

Baylor's experience suggests it is likely that most areas of the country will be affected by the economic forces that encourage the development of integrated health care systems or other mechanisms to deal with these pressures. Second, each system's core processes are likely to vary depending on the system's environment, mission, and values. The act of defining the system's core processes can in itself help a system clarify its vision and mission. It is a valuable learning experience that can be transferred to other areas. Defining core processes can also clarify what functions need to be integrated and which do not. An effort such as the Baylor System Integration Action Team, with its commitment of personnel and other resources, can help increase the visibility and heighten awareness of the integration goals. And the January 1997 target date for completion helps indicate to all the urgency of this effort.

Future Directions at Baylor

As a result of these efforts, Baylor has clarified its mission and developed a strategic vision for the system. However, Baylor's work is by no means finished; in fact, it is just beginning. Baylor continues to face a number of challenges including integrating the community and specialty hospitals into the system, developing information systems, aligning incentives with plans, ensuring that the system has the right pieces for managed care, and developing physician leaders. BHCS needs to build these core processes into a working integrated system. Baylor has undertaken an ambitious effort and only time will tell how successful it will be.

Advocate Health Care

Advocate Health Care has gone through a number of transformations during the course of the study, beginning as Evangelical Health System, then as EHS Health Care, and then merging in January 1995 with Lutheran General HealthSystem to become Advocate. (Hereafter this system will be referred to as EHS Health Care for events up to its merger with Lutheran General; for events following the merger, the system will be referred to as Advocate Health Care.) At the beginning of the study, surveys showed that EHS Health Care perceived itself as somewhat more integrated than the other study systems, especially in regard to human resources, marketing, information systems, and quality assurance. This reflected the amount of effort and attention that EHS leadership had been devoting to functional integration issues. However, the actual level of integration was at best moderate, and it is open to question whether this was true "value-adding" integration or just centralization or standardization.

Obstacles to Integration

Whether this was "true" integration or not was a valid question given the low level of cultural integration characterizing the system at the time. EHS Health Care as a whole was not the focus of many of its members; instead, their focus was on their individual department or, at most, operating unit (for example, the hospital, the home health care agency). This lack of system identification restricted the degree of functional integration that was possible.

A number of other factors also hindered the integration effort. First, understanding of integration and the integration process was not widely distributed. In addition, the hospitals' geographic locations were not conducive to systemwide integration. Finally, the information systems presented a barrier to meaningful integration.

Progress Toward Functional Integration

Often quietly but steadfastly, EHS made strides to become more integrated functionally. Aware of the low cultural integration of the system, EHS leadership gave a great deal of attention to developing an overall system culture that would be infused in all operating units. First, EHS system leaders made a conscious effort to communicate to all employees and boards the system culture and goals, including an understanding of the integration process. EHS established clear, consistent *system* priorities that were communicated to all. Incentives based on achievement of system strategic goals were instituted. Management forums were held to promote system unity. Programs on workplace diversity and changes in the health care field were also initiated.

A major vehicle to promote an EHS culture was the system's CQI/TQM efforts. CQI/TQM training was used to educate people about EHS's mission, central values, and norms. This training was extended deep into the levels of personnel and included lower-level involvement in selection of recipients of awards (for example, co-workers choosing "CQI Stars"). CQI/TQM efforts (for example, meetings, councils, teams, and task forces) were often cross-unit, encouraging interaction among personnel from different operating units and breaking down the operating-unit mentality. Plans were developed to ensure that CQI objectives were aligned with systemwide strategic objectives. Systemwide CQI fairs that featured exhibits, breakout sessions, and information on CQI strategies were held.

The system established EHS University, which offered accredited continuing education programs for nursing, as well as management development and CQI courses. The university was designed to promote the culture, values, and business objectives of the system and to help keep employee skills in alignment with the system's current and future needs. Another system effort to increase system integration, which helped to decrease the hospital focus of the system, was to give EHS hospital CEOs more systemwide responsibilities. In addition, incentives for the top executives were linked to systemwide integration rather than to hospital performance alone. Realizing the limitations that inadequate information systems place on the integration effort, EHS made a concerted effort to build computerized information systems that would link EHS services and units.

Advocate Health Care, created by the merger of EHS and Lutheran General in 1995, has continued to give priority to the development of an organized delivery system. System and physician integration are viewed from conceptual, economic, and clinical perspectives. Conceptual integration occurs through strategic planning that is market based, action oriented, and clearly communicated, and through actions that include development of an Advocate identification, regional management, and physician executives. Given the need to merge two diverse cultures and approaches, to some extent the new system has had to retrace some of its earlier path. Advocate now uses many of the same techniques EHS previously used to promote a common culture. As noted above, EHS system integration was hindered by the lack of geographic coherence of its operating units and was considering development of subregions. Given the breadth of the new Advocate system (eight hospitals and 180 sites throughout the greater Chicago area), Advocate has established a regional management structure. Three regions (North, Central, and South) were created. The small regional leadership teams are housed at the corporate office site to help keep the teams close together and in communication. Finally, Advocate has made a concerted effort to develop physician executives to help link physicians to the system.

Economic integration of Advocate Health Care includes the consolidation of the system financial reports. The assets of the systems have also been merged, and a single governance board has been created. The system is also trying to increase its economic integration with physicians through its management service organization, a "super PHO," and an integrated group practice.

Advocate is also emphasizing the clinical integration of its system, utilizing its culture of TQM and processes of CQI to further not only system integration but also clinical integration. A Clinical Systems Institute was created to help improve clinical processes—and thus the health of the communities that Advocate Health Care serves—by developing clinical guidelines, pathways, and protocols for the full continuum of care across the system.

Keys to Success at Advocate

One of the major reasons for the success of integration efforts at EHS and Advocate has been the commitment of leadership to these efforts. System leaders have made these efforts a priority and have reinforced these priorities with such mechanisms as performance appraisals and reward and incentive systems. They have also emphasized developing a strong culture to provide a platform for integration work. They have put both money and effort into developing clinical and management information systems, viewing them as a foundation for facilitating overall integration efforts. In addition, the new Advocate system board has helped integration efforts by embracing the merger rather than remaining committed to the old systems.

Lessons from the Advocate Experience

The EHS/Advocate experience demonstrates the impact CQI/TQM can have on integration efforts. When adopted properly with a strong commitment, CQI/TQM creates a common approach and language that can be used to develop and enrich a common culture of values. It also helps build integration, because the CQI approach requires interaction of people from different departments and/or operating units, breaking down barriers that hinder integration and building relationships that foster it. The CQI process was so successful at EHS that the system won the 1994 Commitment to Quality Award, sponsored by the Health Care Forum. This strong CQI/TQM effort is not only beneficial for developing a strong systemwide culture and functional integration but also for basing clinical integration initiatives.

Future Directions at Advocate

Advocate continues to see integration as a major challenge of the future. Of primary concern is the "management of diversity." It is trying to deal with the multiple interests of its own members and payers. In addition, Advocate confronts a vast diversity of neighborhoods with widely divergent needs and desires. Reconciling all of these interests will continue to be a problem. Developing more integrated systems of care within each region will also be a continuing challenge as the cultures and practices of the two merging systems continue to evolve.

Franciscan Health System West

Franciscan Health System (FHS), with corporate offices in Aston, Pennsylvania, is a religious-based multiregional health system with operations located on both sides of the country. Franciscan Health

System East has operations in Delaware, Maryland, New Jersey, and Pennsylvania; Franciscan Health System West has operations in the Pacific Northwest, centering in the Washington South Puget Sound region and the eastern Oregon region. Franciscan's religious mission is a central part of its culture with the "values of the Sisters" tying the system together.

Although in study surveys FHS was perceived by its members to be moderately functionally integrated, scoring about the study average, in many respects Franciscan behaved more as a chain of hospitals than as a system or even a set of subsystems. As long as each hospital met its financial targets, it was given much financial and decision-making autonomy. Provision of information to the system was sometimes at the discretion of the individual operating units. The overall good of the system was often not a high priority in operating-unit decision making. Technology assessment and acquisition were primarily left to individual operating units, each making decisions in terms of its own strategic plans and goals. The result was that these decisions often did not support system priorities. Technology acquired at one site was often incompatible even within that one site, let alone across units.

As managed care and health care reform became more prominent in the health care arena, FHS leadership became more concerned about the system's ability to compete. It became obvious that the transcontinental nature of the system limited the type and amount of overall system integration. Even within the two major regions (FHS East and FHS West), geographic distribution of many of the units inhibited integration efforts. As a result, in the early 1990s Franciscan system leadership made the conscious decision to focus system efforts on developing multiple regional organized delivery systems (defined as a patient care delivery system that offers consistent, continuous, and coordinated care across all sites of care) within the overall system. The region with the most immediate potential was the Pacific Northwest, especially the South Sound region. Here the pressures of managed care and health reform were especially strong.

In addition, the system had a concentration of operating units—including three hospitals, a developing physician group, and long-term care facilities—as well as opportunities to expand the breadth and depth of its services through cooperation with other health care providers. Thus, Franciscan's initial efforts to develop a regional integrated delivery system focused on the South Sound region.

Obstacles to Integration

Although FHS had a very strong culture that acted as a glue to hold its components together, it still confronted a number of problems in its efforts to become more functionally integrated. Top leadership may have developed a clear picture of the regional system desired, but for many other people in the system the image was not clear. The plan to develop the organized delivery system followed a long period of FHS cost-reduction efforts that produced nearly $10 million in non-labor savings systemwide and reduced labor costs in Washington by eighty-eight full-time equivalent positions. Anxiety produced by cost-reduction efforts was heightened by a lack of information concerning the reorganization; many wondered what a regional organized delivery system was and what it meant for them and their patient-customers. Franciscan had also been very hospital-oriented in the past. Hospitals often acted independently. Incentives and rewards were hospital based. At times it seemed that the "nonhospital" operating units of the system (for example, physician groups, insurance operating units, home health) were somewhat of an afterthought. Finally, the information systems in the region were inadequate for a fully developed, regionally integrated delivery system.

Progress Toward Functional Integration

Beginning in early 1994, FHS West began a transition to a regional management structure. Even though many people at FHS West were concerned about the stability of their jobs as regionalization and waste reduction occurred, at the same time there was great anticipation of the benefits of regionalization. The collegial, values-driven culture seemed to inspire those affiliated with the system to be willing to sacrifice their jobs in the regional reorganization if this enhanced the care patients received.

The "working definition" model for integration of Franciscan Health System West was driven by the FHS mission, values, and vision that centered around the "moral obligation to improve access, availability, quality and affordability of . . . healthcare services" (Franciscan Health System, 1994). These guiding principles were the basis of system integration efforts that encompassed not only functional integration but also physician and clinical integration, all of which continually reinforced and reshaped one another in an interactive process. The basic design of Franciscan Health System West identified two layers, the West Coast "system" and the regions, for example, the South Puget Sound and Oregon regions. Services and functions would be integrated at the level that seemed most appropriate. Some services and structures could accommodate the whole West Coast system, while others were planned to be implemented only at the regional level.

At the West Coast system level, the position of senior vice president for hospital and health services was created. Integration of system governance was accomplished with the consolidation of the board of trustees. System management was integrated through the consolidation of system and hospital positions. A number of support and ancillary services were shared at the system level.

As mentioned above, at the regional level, the heart of the regional integration effort was and is the South Puget Sound region. The Oregon region, with only two hospitals and little possibility of meaningful integration, shares only management services with the West Coast system. In the South Sound, there has been regional management integration, including the consolidation of administration and management teams into a regional senior management team and a regional management team. Although there are two COOs for the three South Sound hospitals, the senior vice president for hospital and health services has oversight of all three hospitals. Certain functional services are provided or are planned to be provided for the region. Business services provided to the region include patient access and business office activities (including customer services and patient accounting). Financial services such as payroll, accounts payable, budgeting, general accounting, reimbursement, managed care contracting, and decision support are handled at the regional level. Medical records and information management as well as the quality and performance improvement programs are also regional functional services. Other regional functional services include materials management and purchasing; plant, facilities, and master facility planning; dietary and housekeeping product purchasing; risk management and infection control; and mission and ministry services. The regional integration effort extends into the physician and clinical areas, including medical staff integration and pathway development.

Keys to Success at FHS West

A number of environmental or contextual factors have helped promote the efforts of functional integration in the South Sound region. First, managed care is increasingly a major force in the Pacific Northwest; because of this, health care managers, caregivers, and the general public are becoming aware of the changes that need to be made in the health care arena, including the development of more efficient, quality-driven organizations. Washington State health care reform initiatives also prompted changes in the health care institutions, even though many of these initiatives have been at least temporarily abandoned. Second, there is sufficient geographic concentration of both the FHS operating units (hospitals, physician groups, and long-term care units) and the externally owned units and systems (for example, Franciscan and Sisters of Providence formed a joint primary care organization, the Medalia Primary Care Network) with which FHS West could work to develop an integrated health care system.

A third key to FHS West's ability to integrate functionally is its strong values-based culture. Because of this culture, many members of the system have been willing to sacrifice their personal benefit and their operating unit's benefit to the good of the overall regional system and the benefit of the patient. Understanding the importance of the FHS culture, system leadership has acted to ensure that this foundation remains solid in spite of the transformations the system continues to experience. Actions include retreats focusing on the Franciscan heritage, and programs such as a leadership development program entitled "Changes During the Journey," which explained and supported the restructuring efforts. In addition, Franciscan Health System's commitment to values-driven, customer-focused TQM and the dissemination of this approach throughout the system has both augmented the traditional FHS culture and facilitated the integration effort.

Leadership has also been a key factor in the success FHS West has experienced thus far in its integration efforts; leaders have been willing to make some very difficult decisions, especially in terms of cost cutting. What apparently made the cost-reduction and work redesign efforts more palatable to the members of the FHS system was that the changes have been perceived as being carried out in a consistent, equitable, and just manner throughout all units of the system and always with the interests of the patient at their core. This was accomplished in part through the formation by FHS of the interdisciplinary Change Management Work Group, which helped develop restructuring and transition plans that were consistent with the Franciscan values.

Leadership has also implemented mechanisms to help ensure that behavior and actions promote a system perspective and thus system integration. Communication from system leaders to all employees and boards emphasizes system culture, goals, and strategy. Performance appraisal and incentives are increasingly based on system criteria, encouraging employees to consider the good of the system over the good of the individual unit. The creation of a regional senior management position overseeing all three Washington hospitals has reduced the hospital focus of the system. Technology acquisition is based on an assessment process that emphasizes systemwide criteria, not individual operating unit factors. The needs of the regional organized delivery system are now paramount.

Lessons from the FHS Experience

Perhaps the major problem with the integration process at FHS West was the failure of leadership to communicate clearly with the employees throughout the system at the outset their vision of a regional organized delivery system and the plans to achieve this. Regardless of the amount of communication, some anxiety was likely to occur because of the scope of the changes. However, the lack of information produced more anxiety than was probably necessary. As the process proceeded, a more clear vision was presented to the members of the system and the plans gained more acceptance.

The FHS West experience also illustrates the importance of several other factors. First, a strong culture is very helpful when undergoing the often traumatic changes that may occur during the process of integration. Because those who worked for FHS were so committed to the system, they were willing to sacrifice themselves for the good of the system. The FHS West experience also highlights the importance of strong leadership. FHS leaders have had to make some very difficult decisions, but they made the decisions and stood by them. And they have tried to carry out the decisions in as compassionate a manner as possible and thereby gained support for their actions. FHS West leadership also noted that it is helpful to focus at any one time on a few key initiatives rather than to try to accomplish everything at once. And, finally, FHS West shows us that sufficient lead time must be allowed when planning for changes; the preparation and discussion preceding actual implementation can be quite lengthy.

Future Directions at FHS West

Implementation of the regional organized delivery system is planned in two phases: the first emphasizing horizontal integration across the hospitals and the second emphasizing vertical integration across the care continuum. When accomplished, this system will be characterized by common job descriptions, performance criteria, core competencies, and roles. Educational activities will be regionalized, and there will be a standardized information management system with a computerized patient medical record. Treatment in any of the FHS West facilities will be the same high-quality care regardless of where it is delivered. Although a great deal has already been accomplished, FHS continues to face much work as it moves toward its goal of a fully integrated regional delivery system.

Future Challenges and Issues

The functional integration requirements of the organized delivery system of the future are difficult to ascertain because the future health care world that ODSs face is uncertain. First, it is not clear where health care reform will lead; thus, ODSs must plan for a future that may hold unknown governmental requirements. Because the role of the organized delivery system is to provide for the needs of the population(s) that it serves, it is likely that the ODS will also need to change as the needs of the population(s) change. Finally, the changes the ODS will face in the future are likely to increase as technology changes the way medical care is delivered and those who deliver it.

As a result of the potential for change, system integration efforts will need to build in mechanisms that are adaptable rather than static. In fact, the organizational structure of the future is likely to be both fluid and more horizontal than vertical. Nice, clear organizational charts are likely to be replaced by amoeba-like designs that expand, contract, and change shape as the environment dictates. The personnel of these highly fluid systems must be flexible, ambiguity-tolerant individuals. It is likely that those working for the system will hold a number of positions, often in a very short time period. Management is likely to be accomplished through matrix teams, the membership of which will change with the tasks to be accomplished. Both managerial and clinical personnel will need to be multiskilled, both administratively and managerially.

> Some of these changes have been under way for several years involving "total quality management" efforts, reengineering, and business-process redesign. The trend is toward flatter organizations in which managing across has become more critical than managing up and down in a top-heavy hierarchy. . . . In its purest state, the horizontal corporation might boast a skeleton group of senior executives at the top in such traditional support functions as finance and human resources. But virtually everyone else in the organization would work together in multidisciplinary teams that perform core processes, such as product development or sales generation. The upshot: The organization might have only three or four layers of management between the chairman and the staffers in a given process. [Byrne, 1993, pp. 76–77]

With the new organizational design, a number of processes will need to be revamped. This new world of matrix teams and cross-unit, cross-function responsibilities will require new mechanisms for training, evaluation, and compensation. Byrne relates GE's use of "so-called '360-degree appraisal routines' in which peers and others above and below the employee evaluate the performance of an individual in a process. . . . Employees are paid on the basis of the skills they develop rather than merely the individual work they perform" (1993, p. 79).

In summary, the functional requirements of the future are likely to be very different from those of today. First, a system will need to develop the functional support services necessary to manage populations over time. As systems increasingly deal with capitated populations, they will need to develop the support services that allow them to care for these populations longitudinally. The functional infrastructure must also be able to meet the increasing accountability demands. This burden falls most heavily on the information systems and quality management functions of the organization. The functional infrastructure must be able to move from supporting inpatient acute care to primary care and care across the continuum. The functional infrastructure will have to adapt to communication technologies, biomedical science, and work force changes. Finally, the functional infrastructure must simultaneously centralize and decentralize. For example, an ODS must be able to offer a common standard of care across its operating units but also allow for variations in treatments that are dictated by varying conditions. It must assign responsibility for the various functions to whichever levels—be they the system, regional, or operating unit—add the greatest value to the system overall. Functional integration is an ongoing process. However, an organized delivery system must meet the challenges of functional integration in order to promote physician-system and clinical integration. It is to these we turn in Chapters Five and Six.

Physician Integration
Linking Doctors with the System

*What doctor wants to think of his or her goal as fitting
into a system?*

Primary Findings

As described in Chapter Two, physician-system integration is
defined as the extent to which physicians are economically
linked to a system, use its facilities and services, and actively participate in its planning, management, and governance (Gillies and
others, 1993).

This chapter presents some of the primary findings related to
physician-system integration, discusses the challenges involved,
identifies some key success factors based on study systems' experiences, and highlights some future challenges.

Degree of Integration

Table 5.1 highlights some of the more important findings regarding
various economic, administrative, and practice dimensions of physician-system integration in the years 1991 and 1992.

As shown, systems made progress between the two years on a
number of measures. This was particularly true in regard to outpatient visit activity, the percentage of physicians practicing in a system-managed or affiliated practice, the percentage of operating units

Table 5.1. Objective Measures of Physician-System Integration.

Concept or measure	Fiscal year 1991 $\overline{X}$ (Standard deviation; Range)	Fiscal year 1992 $\overline{X}$ (Standard deviation; Range)
Economic involvement		
M.D. utilization activity		
percent accounting for 75+ admissions or outpatient visits	44.2 (11; 34–67)	50.7 (12; 32–76)
percent with 50+ outpatient visits in a system-owned facility	33.0 (28; 2–80)	51.3 (18; 25–83)
percent in a system-managed or affiliated practice	6.6 (7; 0–18)	16.0 (17; 0–42)
Physician benefits		
percent receiving practice management support services	16.6 (22.8; 0–63)	19.0 (18; 0–52)
percent receiving electronic linkage of clinical/financial data	14.7 (21; 0–60)	15.0 (18; 0–52)
Shared contracts		
percent hospital operating units in which hospital-based specialties share contract opportunities	17.1 (15; 0–46)	39.8 (36; 0–100)
Administrative involvement		
percent operating units involving M.D.s in selected set of administrative and governance responsibilities	72.2 (12; 53–89)	69.4 (13; 53–97)

	FY 1991	FY 1992	FY 1994
percent active staff M.D.s paid for administrative responsibilities	6.7 (5; 1–17)		10.0 (9; 0–26)
Physician organization			
IPA (system)			26.0 (38; 0–100)
IPA (independent)			16.9 (26; 0–88)
PHO			15.2 (29; 0–90)
Management service organization			12.1 (22; 0–70)
Foundation			3.2 (9; 0–32)
Other			14.1 (28; 0–100)
System integration			
Perceived physician-system integration (1 = Low; 5 = High)	2.2 (.31; 2–3)	2.3 (.2; 2–3)	2.6 (.2; 2–3)

in which hospital-based specialists (for example, lab, pathology, and radiology) had shared contracts, the percentage of operating units sharing a common medical staff organization, and the percentage of operating units sharing a common physician credentialing process. Increases were more modest regarding practice management support services, administrative and governance involvement of physicians, and the percentage of physicians practicing in groups. There was essentially no change in the percentage of physicians receiving electronic linkage of clinical and financial data. Although not shown, 57 percent of physicians practicing in groups were practicing in groups of fewer than seven physicians.

Physician organizational arrangement data (collected in 1992 only) indicated that study systems were taking a pluralistic approach in working with their physicians. For example, 26 percent of system operating units employed a system-managed or affiliated independent practice association (IPA); 17 percent an independent IPA; 15 percent a physician-hospital organization (PHO); 12 percent an exclusive management service organization (MSO); 11 percent a MSO shared with another entity; and 3 percent used the foundation model (primarily California).

Finally, as shown, perceived physician-system integration changed little between 1991 and 1992. By 1994, however, it had increased to 2.6 (on a 5-point scale where 1 is low and 5 is high), suggesting that system respondents felt they were beginning to make some progress.

Key Relationships

A number of contextual/environmental variables were significantly associated with physician-system integration. For example, systems that developed more internally rather than through merger and acquisition were *less likely* to involve physicians in management and governance. As discussed elsewhere, this was primarily due to problems posed by "cash cow" hospitals that were frequently reluctant to give up their established relationships with physicians in order to promote systemwide integration initiatives (Shortell, Gillies, and others, 1993).

Adopting a prospector strategic orientation emphasizing innovation and risk taking was positively associated with greater physician involvement. This is because developing new programs and services, signing managed care contracts, and taking on more of the risk requires greater physician involvement in management and governance of a delivery system, given the close relationships among benefit design, care provision, and financial solvency.

Other key findings included the following:

- Systems that developed more internally were less likely to have a common medical staff organization or shared credentialing.

- Systems with a prospector strategic orientation were more likely to have higher percentages of physicians practicing in groups.

- A greater degree of HMO market penetration was positively associated with a greater percentage of physicians practicing in groups.

- The greater the distance between a system's hospitals, the smaller the percentage of physicians practicing in groups.

- The greater the degree of standardization of support functions and policies (for example, human resources, strategic planning financial policies, information systems, and quality assurance), the greater the degree of physician-system integration, particularly in regard to physician participation in management.

- A greater degree of physician-system integration (for example, shared medical staff organization, common credentialing, and physicians practicing in groups) was positively associated with greater total system revenue and greater cash flow.

Two findings deserve comment. First, we found that the depth of services offered by a system was positively associated with physician-system integration, particularly in regard to physicians practicing in groups of twenty-five or more. This finding suggests that when certain services (for example, cardiovascular, oncology) are provided at multiple sites, incentives may be created for greater physician-system integration in order to better coordinate care at the multiple sites. Second, contrary to our prediction, the degree of *perceived* functional integration of the system was largely unrelated to physician-system integration and was actually inversely related to the percentage of physicians practicing in groups. This finding suggests the possibility that systems with *fewer* physicians practicing in groups may have greater need for functional integration in such areas as information systems, quality management, human resource, marketing, and planning because these are needed to support physicians who are largely practicing solo or in small partnerships. It may also be the case that in those systems with more physicians practicing in groups, many of the management support functions may be contained within the group itself. In this sense group practice may *substitute* to some degree for functional integration as measured at the system level.

We also examined physician-system integration at the level of the individual hospitals within the study systems. The key findings here were as follows:

- The longer the hospital had been with the system, the less likely it was to have a common medical staff with another hospital in the system and the less likely it was to share credentialing processes.

- Hospitals that were a part of larger systems were less likely to be integrated with their physicians.

- Hospitals with a group-oriented culture (for example, one emphasizing participation, involvement, affiliation, and support [Quinn and Kimberly, 1984]) enjoyed a greater degree of physician-system integration.

- A greater degree of perceived quality assurance integration was positively associated with a greater degree of physician-system integration.

The latter three findings suggest that as systems become larger, it becomes more difficult to foster a group-oriented culture (Shortell and others, 1995a); as a result, greater problems of physician-system integration may occur. At the same time, quality assurance and CQI/TQM approaches may act as positive factors in helping to promote greater physician-system integration (Shortell and others, 1995a).

In regard to individual hospital financial performance, we found that when a greater percentage of a hospital's physicians were practicing in groups and were active users of the system, there was also:

- Greater total revenue per adjusted patient day

- Greater net patient revenue per adjusted patient day

- Greater total cash flow

- Greater net cash flow

With the exception of functional integration, the above findings are generally supportive of the hypotheses outlined in Chapter Three regarding the influence of the contextual and market/environmental variables on physician-system integration. Market pressure in the form of HMO and related managed care activities provides the incentive to develop closer relationships with physicians; such system characteristics as historical development, strategic orientation, and size can serve as facilitators or barriers to forging such integration. It is also important to recognize certain changes occurring within medicine itself.

Medicine: A Profession in Transition

To understand the difficulties associated with forging new relationships with physicians, it is helpful to briefly highlight the changes occurring within the profession itself. A common theme has been the increased dependence of physicians on organizations to achieve their professional objectives (Freidson, 1970a, 1970b; Scott, 1982; Starr, 1983; and Stevens, 1971). In recent years, the growing pressure of managed care and the movement away from the hospital as the center of the delivery system (Shortell, Gillies, and Devers, 1995) have caused further strains on traditional relationships between physicians and health care organizations. Managed care pressures have caused physicians (and other health care professionals) to become involved in utilization management practices; the development of guidelines, protocols, and pathways; participation in quality improvement project teams; and development of clinical outcome, functional health status, and patient satisfaction measures. Many of these activities have required physicians to work in teams, something for which most are ill prepared, given the medical school emphasis on individual clinical experience and patient responsibility, as well as the probable self-selection of individuals into the profession who prefer to work alone and who prize their autonomy.

The trend away from the hospital as the center of the delivery system has had an equally important impact on the profession. The growth of technology that can be used in outpatient settings has facilitated growth in the delivery of outpatient services. For example, outpatient visits grew 73 percent between 1980 and 1992

(American Hospital Association, 1993b), and ambulatory surgery as a percentage of all surgeries approximates 70 percent (American Hospital Association, 1993b). In the San Francisco Bay area, 75 percent of AIDS patients are treated and cared for exclusively on an outpatient basis from diagnosis to death. In addition, financial pressures to control costs have resulted in the growth of more care in physicians' offices, at home, and almost any place other than the acute inpatient unit of the hospital. As a result, there has been tremendous interest in the growth of primary care networks and physician group practice. For example, in the Minneapolis–St. Paul market, the percentage of physicians practicing in groups increased from 58 percent in 1979 to 95 percent in 1993, with a nearly five-fold increase in the percentage of larger groups of over twenty-five full-time equivalent physicians (Kralewski and Wingert, 1995). Over the same time period, the percentage of multispecialty groups grew from 21 percent to 36 percent. This has led to (1) a splintering or strain in the relationship between primary care physicians and specialists as primary care physicians play a more central role in securing and allocating patients and (2) a diminution of the role of the organized hospital medical staff as the vehicle for physician influence within an organizational context—in favor of new economic arrangements such as PHOs, MSOs, foundations, and large multispecialty practices. These changes disrupt established norms, values, and behaviors of all parties, creating challenges that are similar to attempting to build a new house in the midst of an earthquake. Some of the tremors associated with building the new relationships are discussed below.

Barriers and Challenges to Integration

The obstacles to forming closer physician-system partnerships can be divided into those that are largely external to the organization and those that are primarily internal. The external are less susceptible to the direct influence or control of the organization than are the internal. The external factors will primarily require changes in public policy.

External Factors

The two primary external factors influencing physician-system integration are the lack of common financial incentives and the presence of various legal and regulatory barriers.

Lack of Common Economic Incentives

In most parts of the United States, hospitals and physicians do not experience the same financial incentives; this is due to the variety of forms of payment, including per diem, per case, fee-for-service, discounted fee-for-service, salaried arrangements, and so on. Conflicting incentives were a particular problem for systems with some physicians in salaried group practice models and others in various fee-for-service models. These payment modes in turn may exist under varying degrees of capitation, ranging from full capitation of the entire delivery system to capitation of individual parts to no capitation. Even the federal Medicare program with its separation of Part A (hospital payment) and Part B (physician payment) acts as a major barrier to closer relationships between physicians, hospitals, and overall systems of care (Hurley, 1993). These frequently conflicting financial incentives get in the way of the best of intentions and undermine relationships that are already based on a shaky ground of trust. The role that private market forces, state health initiatives, and federal policy play in this regard is discussed in Chapter Eight.

Legal and Regulatory Barriers

Efforts at physician-system integration can be also impeded by state and federal laws and regulations. Some states such as California, for example, prohibit hospital ownership of medical groups. Also, tax-exempt financing guidelines may prohibit exceeding 20 percent physician membership on corporate health system boards. In addition, federal antitrust legislation if applied inflexibly can prohibit mergers and consolidations of physician groups and of physician groups with hospitals and other health care entities. While these issues are not a major focus of this book, they are clearly constraints that must be dealt with by those attempting to achieve higher levels of physician-system integration.

Internal Factors

Internal obstacles to physician-system integration include satisfaction with the status quo, fear and distrust, tensions between primary care physicians and specialists, the need to form a greater number of physician groups, the relative lack of physician leadership, and relatively weak clinical and financial information systems.

Satisfaction with the Status Quo

Many physicians throughout the United States do not see the need for significant change because they are still doing relatively well financially and are meeting their professional goals. This is particularly true for physicians with established practices and for physicians practicing in the Stage 1 unstructured "access" markets. While they are generally aware of the pressures for cost containment and the growth of managed care, they do not believe it will come to their area or affect them personally. Even in Stage 2 and Stage 3 markets, there are pockets of physician resistance among those who have somehow managed to escape the advancing managed care glacier. As we will discuss, the leader's job in such a situation is to make physicians uncomfortable, then manage that discomfort and channel the anxieties and fears into constructive action: a challenging task.

Fear and Distrust

Even those physicians who are dissatisfied with the status quo and have recognized the need for significant change are frequently immobilized by fear and distrust. Some of this is generalized fear and distrust related to perceived loss of clinical and practice autonomy and a general inability to control or influence their professional careers. Some of it is a fear of large organizations. Other aspects of their fear and distrust are more specifically related to the degree of trust existing between and among physicians, hospitals, and other entities constituting the local delivery system. For example, at several systems, physicians in small partnerships and group practices feared that the large multispecialty group practices within the system would, in effect, force their practices and policies on the smaller groups of physicians and, in effect, take away their patients. In other cases, physicians feared that data on patient outcomes would be used against them.

It is important to recognize that, in many respects, the local voluntary community hospital has been the physicians' "organizational security blanket," serving as the forum for exercising their professional autonomy in a collective fashion. As more health care services are delivered outside of hospitals and as financial pressures continue to push in that direction, hospitals are no longer the focal point for the organization of the delivery system. This has served to increase physicians' fears and anxieties as they search for new organizational homes to protect their interests—for example, multispecialty group practices, PHOs, MSOs, and related arrangements. In the process they are finding that many of these arrangements are based on economic, legal, and managerial parameters (in addition to clinical parameters) with which they are unfamiliar—thus promoting more anxiety. In the present study, the difficulty of integrating physicians into the overall system was particularly pronounced for those systems in which key hospitals still enjoyed significant autonomy; such autonomy reinforced physician linkages with the hospital rather than with the system (Shortell, Gillies, and others, 1993).

The willingness of physicians to accept at-risk contracts often serves as a litmus test for assessing the degree of fear and distrust existing within a given system. Physicians frequently pass through seven stages before feeling comfortable enough to go at-risk. The physician begins with a general lack of awareness: "I don't know what you are talking about." Next comes denial: "I don't believe you," or "It won't happen here." Anger: "If you had run this system right, we wouldn't have been placed in this situation." The fourth stage is characterized by conflict over what to do; next comes resignation and acceptance: "We don't like it, but we will have to deal with it." Stage six is curiosity: "I wonder how it might work?" Finally, the physician is willing to at least accept some small fee discounts (Shalowitz, 1994). Depending on the degree of managed care pressure in the marketplace and the degree of competition from other physicians and systems, the next step is to accept some risk-bearing contracts.

Conflict Between Primary Care Physicians and Specialists

There are "naturally occurring" differences between primary care physicians and specialists (as well as within these two groups) as a function of career interests, educational experiences, preferences for different kinds of patients, and related factors. The current economic environment intensifies these differences as primary care physicians and specialists see themselves competing for patients while trying to change practice styles in the process. More important, the relative power of specialists has diminished as primary care physicians have assumed a more central role as the initial contact point with patients and as major decision makers regarding referrals to specialists and sites of care throughout the system. This relative power shift is accentuated by a shortage of primary care physicians in some cases and a rather marked oversupply of specialists in nearly all cases. For example, although only one-third of the nation's physicians are primary care physicians, in some of the more aggressive managed care markets there is need for a physician base composed of at least 50 to 60 percent primary care physicians. In a number of markets, the required size of a viable primary care physician network is beyond many delivery system expectations and can require capital of up to $16 million (Advisory Board Company, 1993, p. xiv). Understandably, specialists are concerned about this redeployment of capital and attention to primary care physicians and away from specialty care.

Given this situation, systems face a tough challenge in attempting to bring primary care physicians and specialists together to accept risk. The issues involve how the capitated dollar will be divided, criteria for patient referral, the appropriate use of protocols, pathways, and outcome measures, and the respective role of primary physicians and specialists in managing chronic illness. Systems such as Baylor, which have had a traditionally strong emphasis on specialty care, face particular challenges, as evidenced by the following exchange:

PRIMARY CARE PHYSICIAN: The majority of the patient population has to be seen by a primary care physician. For a while, specialists dominated health care, but now there is a move back to medicine based on primary care. Specialists are now seen as spending money, whereas before they were seen as earning money (for a hospital or system).

SPECIALIST: I don't like it. The situation may actually change under capitation where individual physicians would become their own gatekeepers.

PRIMARY CARE PHYSICIAN: But entry into the system will continue to come through the primary care physician.

Too Few Groups

As managed care pressures grow, there is likely to be a significant increase in the percentage of physicians practicing in groups. There are many reasons for this but among the most important are (1) to achieve sufficient breadth of coverage across a given geographic market and avoid being locked out of contracts; (2) to better coordinate patient care and provide more cost-effective care through the development of protocols, pathways, and related means; (3) to spread practice overhead costs; (4) to improve communication among physicians and other caregivers; (5) to transfer learning more quickly; (6) to develop a culture that promotes teamwork; and (7) to develop a sufficiently large patient base upon which to collect reliable and valid functional health status, patient outcome, and patient satisfaction data. Groups can also increase physicians' sense of control over their professional careers and provide some degree of psychological security. But many of these possible advantages are future oriented and relatively intangible, which means that encouraging physicians to practice in groups and, beyond that, encouraging small groups to form larger groups, is a challenging task.

Lack of Physician Leadership

Initiating and implementing the changes required to deal with the turbulent forces in the health care environment require concerted leadership from all parties. In this regard, physician leadership has frequently been a missing link in the health care chain (Hughes, 1994). Most physicians, understandably, are interested in practicing medicine and, generally, have a distaste for administrative or managerial concerns. However, as professional work is increasingly practiced in complex organizations enmeshed in turbulent environments, there is a need for professionals to assume broader leadership and managerial roles. The first generation of physician leaders generally received little management training and focused their attention primarily on individual institutions, departments, or divisions. Typical examples were the hospital vice president for medical affairs, the director of medical education, or the chief of a specific service line or division.

A second generation of physician leadership is beginning to emerge that focuses on a broader range of health care delivery. These physicians are beginning to receive more systematic training. They are assuming systemwide responsibility for clinical integration, quality improvement, and group practice management (Dunham, Kindig, and Schulz, 1994). Their training ranges from short, two- to four-day intensive courses to summer courses to, in some cases, M.B.A.s and related master's degrees in health services management. These individuals must overcome significant obstacles to become effective executives, not the least of which is their "marginality" in terms of being neither fully accepted by their colleagues—who will view them as having sold out to administration—nor fully accepted by their nonclinical managerial colleagues, who may view them as intruders or Johnny-come-latelies.

There is need, however, for a third generation of leadership in which all physicians in medical school and residency programs would learn some basic managerial and leadership skills in communication, conflict management, change management, team building, and continuous improvement methodologies in order to be better prepared to practice in a changed environment and better prepared to accept as well as contribute to new leadership approaches. A subgroup of these physicians will need to choose clinical careers that combine medicine and management in helping to restructure the delivery system.

Poorly Implemented Integrated Information Systems

A major operational barrier to physician-system integration is the lack of information systems that connect patients and providers across the different settings of care. These systems are needed not only to provide access, cost, quality, and outcome data for external accountability purposes but also to meet continuous quality improvement objectives. The exchange of information is at the center of the physician-patient relationship and yet, relative to other fields, health care spends little on this fundamental process—it constitutes slightly less than 2 percent of operating budgets versus 6 to 7 percent in other fields (Dorenfest, 1995). But money alone is not the answer. Caregivers and managers need to do a better job of delineating what the information is for, what type of information is most useful, and how the information can best be turned into *knowledge* and indeed *wisdom* in serving patient and community needs.

Influence of Market Maturity

The external and internal barriers to physician-system integration discussed above tend to vary as a function of the degree of market maturity, as shown in Table 5.2.

Table 5.2. Barriers to Physician-System Integration by Stages of Market Maturity.

Barriers	Stage 1 Unstructured "access" market	Stage 2 "Loose cost" market	Stage 3 Consolidated "advanced cost" market	Stage 4 Strict managed care "value" market
Lack of common economic incentives	++	++	+	0
Legal and regulatory barriers	++	+	+	+
Satisfaction with status quo	0	++	++	+
Fear and distrust	0	++	++	++
Primary care physicians versus specialists	0	++	++	+
Physician group practice formation issues	0	++	++	+
Physician leadership issues	++	++	++	+
Information system issues	0	++	++	++

Note: ++ = significant barrier; + = barrier; 0 = usually not a barrier or factor.

In the Stage 1 unstructured "access" market, major barriers include the lack of common economic incentives to initiate action, satisfaction with the status quo, and lack of physician leadership. In Stage 1, providers and systems are only beginning to realize that the world may be changing.

In the Stage 2 "loose cost" market, characterized by growing managed care pressures, conflict begins to emerge around the formation of physician group practices (who is in and who is out), the growing influence of primary care physicians relative to specialists, fear and distrust of system management and of large medical groups, and legal and regulatory barriers that inhibit or prohibit various structures and arrangements. These issues are further complicated by the Stage 1 barriers of the mixed economic and payment systems and the lack of physician leadership to deal with the problems.

In the Stage 3 consolidated "advanced cost" market, in which there exists a critical mass of systems and networks competing for the managed care dollar, the economic incentives begin to align and satisfaction with the status quo largely disappears. Ongoing fear and distrust, physician group practice formation, legal and regulatory barriers, primary care versus specialist battles, and ongoing physician leadership issues take center stage. At this point the inability to meet the accountability demands of purchasers due to inadequate information systems also emerges.

Finally, in the Stage 4 "value" market, the major challenges remaining include the conflict between primary care physicians and specialists regarding referrals and distribution of the capitated dollar, ongoing legal and regulatory barriers to structuring new relationships, and the need to upgrade information systems. In Stage 4 markets, systems may also still be experiencing problems with ongoing fear and distrust and with forming or consolidating physician groups, and some need for additional physician leadership. The biggest barrier in Stage 4 is not shown: the need to develop a more clinically integrated continuum of care. This vital issue is addressed in Chapter Six.

Key Success Factors and Some Best Practices

The speed with which physician-system integration might proceed is driven by two major groups of factors: the external environment demanding change and the internal capabilities of the organization to manage change. The study findings as well as experiences in other markets throughout the United States (Alexander, Burns, and Zuckerman, 1995) suggest that physician-system integration is further along in those markets with greater HMO and managed care penetration and in areas with a greater number of competing systems. While the external environmental forces are a necessary condition for integration, they are insufficient by themselves. Based on the present intensive study of the eleven systems, more casual observation of other systems, and review of existing literature, we have identified the following seven key success factors for physician-system integration: (1) creating a zone of "manageable discomfort"; (2) communicating the vision and selling the strategy; (3) empowering physicians; (4) providing incentives; (5) using pluralistic partnership approaches and models; (6) forming more group practices; and (7) providing the necessary information system and infrastructure support. Each of these is discussed below.

Creating a Zone of "Manageable Discomfort"

An important barrier to changing any organization or social system is people who are satisfied with the existing state. Getting physicians to recognize the need to change their practices as a function of the changing economic, technological, and social forces is particularly difficult in Stage 1 and Stage 2 markets. The leader's job is to create the right amount of discomfort—to create sufficient dissatisfaction with the status quo to get people to try new approaches while at the same time providing a sense of security and reassurance that the new approaches will pay off and will, indeed, result in achieving the desired vision. Change that is seen as too abrupt, too radical, or unachievable often results in overreaction and negative "acting out" behavior that can pose a bigger threat to the organization than if no change were attempted at all. Thus, the trick is to create a zone of manageable discomfort.

In the systems studied, leaders did several things to create such a zone. For example, they would frequently point to what was happening in other markets throughout the country. They would bring in physician leaders from those markets to speak at medical staff meetings. Leaders would also organize trips for key physicians to visit other systems where changes were being successfully implemented. Leaders would continually expose physicians to data on their own local market and what competitors were doing. A number of systems, such as Advocate, Baylor, Franciscan, Sharp, and Sutter, developed their own managed care product or shared an ownership position in such a product in order to signal to their physicians the importance of learning how to practice more cost-effective care in a managed care environment and to gain some experience in doing so.

In order to increase the comfort level and the ability to deal with the changes, the systems also invested in extensive physician leadership development programs, managed care "colleges," and support units to assist in conducting clinical outcome studies. Most significant, these systems spent tens of millions of dollars for upgrading clinical and management information systems. In doing so, the study systems also learned that creating a zone of manageable discomfort was not a one-time effort; the zone had to be continuously monitored and maintained even in the more mature markets. This was accomplished by being very sensitive to managing the pace of change, knowing when to speed it up and, perhaps even more important, when to slow it down. For example, a major change initiated at UniHealth was to involve physicians in consolidating eleven hospital labs into one that would serve the entire system in a cost-effective fashion. As expected, numerous issues arose generating considerable conflict. But the process was well managed by an astute executive who could sense when things were moving too fast or when there was too much uneasiness, and would respond by taking the issue "off the table" and letting it percolate on the back burner.

Only when the parties involved had a chance to regain their momentum and comfort level with each other and again saw the need to address the issue would it be brought back into the discussion. Savvy, experienced leadership and management is needed to strike the right chords of creative tension.

Communicating the Vision—Selling the Strategy

As for any professional, the primary interest of physicians is in their own career. Organizations are seen as vehicles for advancement of their careers. In the past, the hospital has been the primary vehicle for advancement of most physician's careers. Many physicians—particularly specialists—perceive the move toward the creation of more integrated delivery systems across the continuum of care as diminishing the central role of the hospital, their primary source of organizational identity. Thus they are looking for new anchors lest they be cast adrift on the surging waters of managed care. Systems must respond by communicating the vision of an organized delivery system in a way that engages positive physician behavior. Recent evidence suggests that physicians identify with systems that are perceived to be attractive and that have a positive external image (Dukerich, Golden, and Shortell, 1995). System identification was, in turn, related to physician cooperative behaviors. This means that the system vision must be communicated in a way that addresses the physician's economic and professional needs for security, growth, a reasonable degree of autonomy, and a sense of control over his or her own destiny. As we will discuss, this involves empowerment, incentives, and pluralistic partnership models. But it must begin with a clearly articulated, focused strategy of what the system is about and what the physician's role is within the strategy. The strategy must then be communicated and sold at every opportunity (Hambrick and Cannella, 1989).

Based on the present study, systems that pursued a prospector or analyzer strategy were significantly further along in physician-system integration than those systems that were pursuing more of a defender strategy. Defenders would, for example, continue to emphasize acute inpatient care and view the hospital as the center of the system. It is not surprising that physician-system integration would be more advanced among those systems that have adopted prospector or analyzer strategies because executing such a strategy depends critically on physician involvement. Related research has also highlighted the importance of physician-system integration to market expansion and growth objectives (Alexander, Burns, and Zuckerman, 1995).

Most of the systems studied were in the process of making the transition from being largely hospital focused to becoming more physician centered. These included strategies to expand primary care networks, add services missing in the continuum of care, tie physicians closer to the system, cut costs, reduce duplication, and invest in an information infrastructure that would produce reliable and valid data on quality and outcome of care. In varying degrees, more physicians were involved in making and implementing these decisions. Physician leaders who helped to formulate those same strategies were increasingly involved in communicating them. In several systems, strategic planning was centered around physician groups rather than the hospitals. These groups and their related organizations, not the hospital's medical staff organization, were the central communication forum. Frequent use was made of retreats, special task forces, and educational forums for communicating and selling the strategy. At the same time, almost all systems recognized the need to do a better job of communicating and selling the strategy. As expressed by one system respondent:

> We don't communicate well because of the size and the culture. Administrators and the physicians do their jobs and communicate only what is necessary to the other party. Historically, the two groups have peacefully co-existed. This is not good enough now. The grapevine is not good enough to deal with communication. Change is too fast paced, and the grapevine can spread rumors that raise anxiety.

Empowering Physicians

In a world characterized by increasing paradox (Handy, 1989), perhaps the ultimate paradox in health care is the need to empower physicians. As one of the most dominant groups in the history of the professions (Begun and Lippincott, 1993; Freidson, 1970a, 1970b; Starr, 1983; and Stevens, 1971), how is it that physicians need to be empowered? The answer lies in the recognition that most physicians are at a comparative disadvantage in dealing with the financial, managerial, and organizational issues associated with the delivery of health care in the late 1990s. These issues have largely been addressed by a growing cadre of health services executives trained in health services administration programs within schools of public health and business schools, as well as by executives from other industries who have been recruited into health care. Historically, there has been a relative separation of medicine and management, with the voluntary medical staff and related mechanisms serving as the primary forums for resolving problems and differences. But economic, political, and social forces are pushing strongly for a marked increase in the interdependence of medicine and management while at the same time disrupting the established structures used in the past. The new relationships and the issues associated with them are now discussed in *economic units* involving group practices, IPAs, PHOs, MSOs, and related models that attempt to create incentives for concerted action. As the transformation of health care increasingly focuses on reorganizing the way patient care is delivered, the physicians' expertise and experience grow in importance. Physicians possess important knowledge that nonclinical health care executives do not: of what services should be offered; what conditions or disease states are amenable to developing clinical service lines; what diagnoses and conditions are most amenable for developing guidelines, protocols, and pathways; what clinical outcome measures can be reliably and validly developed; how new technology is likely to influence treatment patterns; and of other related issues. The bridge between "administrative" and "clinical" decision making has been largely abolished. This need for greater clinical input combined with the physicians' need to control their own destiny has created the imperative for greater physician empowerment.

Two factors are essential for empowerment to work. First, those being empowered must have the competencies and capabilities necessary to carry out the tasks delegated to them and be motivated to do so. It does little good and some might argue much harm to empower people who are largely unable to execute what they are being empowered to do. In brief, *empowerment* means not only to delegate but to provide people with the *power* (that is, training, tools, and so on) to succeed. Second, for empowerment to work, those in positions of authority and leadership must be willing to "let go" and share some of their authority with others. This is difficult for those with a high need for control, who need to be perceived as a hero or heroine (Bradford and Cohen, 1984), and who have primarily exercised leadership through the position of their formal office. It is particularly difficult in health care organizations, where there may be distrust between executives and physicians (Shortell, 1991; Alexander, Burns, and Zuckerman, 1995). Physicians and health care executives have to earn each other's trust. More physicians have to be prepared to pick up the leadership reins and educate themselves regarding the financial, managerial, and organizational issues associated with modern health care delivery. At the same time, health care executives must be willing to invest in developing capable physician leaders and must themselves be willing to let go of the reins and share power with physicians.

What are systems doing to empower physicians? They are transforming their cultures, expanding their educational programs, increasing physician involvement, and aligning incentives.

Culture

Most systems are working hard to create more group-oriented cultures emphasizing teamwork, cooperation, sharing of information, and developing pride in the organization. The following comments of Fairview physicians are illustrative.

"Fairview is a fair organization. They are as good as their word. . . . They are willing to go that extra mile."

"One of the positive points is that administration listens and tries to help physicians."

"A positive aspect of the culture is the way that [Fairview] responds to situations. Physicians feel empowered."

Education

Every study system either already had or has since instituted an ongoing physician leadership development program. As expressed by executives at Advocate Health System (formerly EHS Health Care and Lutheran General HealthSystem): "The EHS vision puts physicians in leadership roles recognizing that they are the gate-keepers and true integrators of health care" (Risk and Francis, 1994).

Although some physicians volunteered for these programs, most were carefully selected to represent different specialties, age groups, and areas of interest. The programs ranged from two- and three-day intensive seminars on selected topics to an integrated curriculum spread across one year or more. Most systems, such as Advocate, Sharp, and Sutter, conduct their programs in conjunction with local universities, whereas some, such as Henry Ford, primarily use internal resources. Some systems include nonclinical executives in their programs to provide them with exposure to clinical epidemiology, decision analysis, and protocol and pathway development. In some systems, as many as four hundred physicians have received such leadership training. Experience suggests that investment in physician leadership development is likely to have high payoff: increased physician commitment to the system, and increased physician willingness and ability to actively participate in new shared ownership arrangements such as PHOs and in overall management and governance responsibilities. Having greater numbers of trained physician leaders does not mean that physicians, hospitals, and other components of the delivery system will operate without conflict, differences, or moments of distress but rather that these difficulties will be more directly addressed with data where it is available and with a more sophisticated set of skills and understandings. Henry Ford's approach to physician leadership development (discussed in Chapter Six) illustrates many of these points.

Involvement

During the period of the study there was also a significant increase in the meaningful involvement of physicians in the management and governance of the system. This was reflected not only in increasing numbers of physicians serving on governing boards and assuming key management positions (such as the vice president for clinical affairs or the vice president for clinical integration) but also in their intermingling throughout the system on task forces, committees, quality improvement project teams, and related forums. Evidence suggests that such involvement is positively associated with operational performance (Molinari, Alexander, Morlock, and Lyles, 1995). Further, several systems have centered their strategic planning process around physician groups rather than hospitals. Sentara has reorganized its entire management structure, creating an eight-person management council with four of the eight being physicians. This council is charged with guiding the system's overall strategic direction.

Incentives

Why should physicians align themselves with a given system? While there may be many reasons, certainly a dominant one is economic incentives. Simply put, physicians are likely to align themselves with those systems that can help physicians maintain and expand their practices in an environment characterized by increased financial risk. For example, a recent examination by J. Shalowitz, M.D. (1993) revealed what primary care physicians want a health care system to do:

- Have a sufficient volume of patients to diffuse risk, or use creative payment schedules until the risk targets are met

- Provide timely and accurate eligibility data, preferably through on-line computer linkages

- Set capitation based on realistic risks and allow compensation for adverse selection

- Provide appropriate stop-loss insurance and first dollar re-insurance—the latter for high-risk cases such as open heart, psych and chemical dependency

- Help obtain favorable supplier contracts using the system's market-share power—for example, to purchase packages and obtain aggressive specialists' contracts

- Enable the physician to do his or her own benefit interpretations

- Leave the physician alone to manage his or her own business—that is, do not micro-manage care

- Share profits as befits a true partnership

Based on the experience of the study systems, we would add that physicians want assistance in conducting clinical outcome studies to improve care and to be provided with outcome data for purposes of external reporting.

As to sharing profits, models whereby physicians become shareholders in their practices provide an incentive to work for the long-term growth of the practice. Many groups affiliated with the study systems also used short-term financial incentives such as incentive pay above and beyond a base salary contingent on meeting productivity *and* patient satisfaction objectives. Systems were also increasingly paying physicians for undertaking a variety of administrative tasks and responsibilities. For example, Advocate, Baylor, Fairview, and Sharp all had policies of compensating physicians for efforts on behalf of the system that detracted from their practice time. Fairview, for example, pays physicians for board participation at the rate of

$3,000 per year and for the development of protocols, guidelines, pathways, and outcome measures at $2,500 per year. Systems such as Baylor and Sentara pay physicians $100 per meeting for participation and for work on process reengineering and protocol development. Still others, such as Sisters of Providence, compensate physicians for time spent beyond four hours at any one time or event.

The importance and effectiveness of economic and related incentives is expressed in the following comments of Baylor physicians.

"Sharing the benefits of partnership will only happen if a system is integrated financially and economically. . . . The more economically aligned incentives are, the better it will be."

"Physicians need to be made part of the 'team'—possibly through joint ventures in having a financial stake in the activities. In the past Baylor maintained physician loyalty by excellence in high technology. . . . In the future, it won't be possible to do that so that the only way to make physicians loyal is to make them part of the team."

Pluralistic Approaches and Models

Theoretically, salaried and equity models of physician-system relationships would appear to best promote physician-system integration. But the experience of the participating systems suggests that those offering a *variety of physician partner relationships simultaneously* were furthest along in their integration efforts as measured by the indicators discussed in Chapter Three. The underlying logic is to work with physicians "where they are" in terms of their age, experience, stage of their career, specialty, preferences, and related variables. Thus, systems such as Sharp, Sutter, and UniHealth would typically have loosely organized IPAs existing side by side with open PHOs, closed PHOs, MSOs, foundation models, and equity models. It is significant to note that this pluralism existed in highly penetrated Stage 4 managed care markets such as Minneapolis, Northern California, Los Angeles, and San Diego. Henry Ford Health System, occupying a less penetrated Stage 2 market (Detroit), uses a salaried multispecialty group practice model as its primary form of partnership. Thus, it is *not* the case that there is necessarily a logical progression from loose models to tight models as one goes from Stage 1 to Stage 4 markets. This observation is also supported by a recent study of physician-organization arrangements in four other systems, where it was found that salaried integrated models were prevalent among all four systems including those in the early stages of managed care penetration (Alexander, Burns, and Zuckerman, 1995). But it does appear to be the case that in more heavily penetrated managed care markets, a greater percentage of physicians will be in more integrated arrangements such as closed panel PHOs, salaried, and equity models. It is simply that the other more loosely organized models do not go away. These more loosely organized models might be viewed as "collectors of physicians" that give physicians experience in providing care under various at-risk arrangements. As managed care pressures grow and the need for more cost-effective practice increases, and as physician leadership matures, many of these physicians see the need for more integrated models such as the foundation, salaried, and equity models (Schultz, Napiewocki, and Nerenz, 1994). The extent to which this occurs critically depends on the extent to which physicians believe they can exert sufficient influence and control over the partnership.

While all models appear to exist in all markets in nearly all systems, various characteristics of physician partnering can be placed on a continuum of less to more advanced in terms of their integration potential. This is shown in Figure 5.1.

The important point to note is that the various organizational structures (IPAs, PHOs, MSOs, and so on) tend to be associated with various practices designed to restructure and better integrate patient care. For example, very little care restructuring occurs in the "getting started" stage. The primary focus of activity at this stage is in getting physicians together through IPA formation and encouraging group practice development. Patient care restructuring begins to occur in the "moving forward" stage as more formalized support

Figure 5.1. Physician Partner Relationships and Physician-System Integration Potential.

Getting started →	Moving forward →	Taking off
Independent practice associations (IPAs)	Physician-hospital organizations (PHOs)	Salaried, staff models
Encouraging group practice formation	Management service organizations (MSOs)	Equity models
• Education	Foundation models	Widespread clinical applications of continuous quality improvement
• Site visits	Group practice consolidation	Mature outcomes management system combines protocols, clinical outcomes, functional health status, and patient satisfaction measures
• Development funds	Develop clinical protocols	
• Practice subsidization	Begin outcomes management system	
• Practice acquisition	Develop automated medical record	Use automated medical record
Discounted fee-for-service arrangements	Accept partial at-risk contracts	Develop population-based, continuum of care, community health status measures
		Accept full-risk contracts

services are provided to physicians who are increasingly practicing in groups. It is at this stage that one begins to observe the development of clinical protocols, outcome management systems, and common medical records, as providers begin to take on the responsibility of some at-risk contracting. These activities accelerate in the "taking off" stage, where more physicians are practicing in salaried staff and equity models and are accepting full at-risk contracts. These provide the incentives for development of a mature outcome management system and widespread clinical applications of CQI/TQM.

As previously mentioned, those systems in the "taking off" stage will still typically have "getting started" and "moving forward" components as well. The glue that holds the varied approaches and activities together is the systems' strategy, vision, culture, and physician leadership development programs. Certain practices serve as implementation steps to achieve effective partnerships. The most important of these steps are outlined below:

- Make *quality of health care* the overarching goal of all partners, a goal that everyone can buy into.

- Develop and maintain a culture that gives priority to *professional competence* and performance of all parties involved in the partnership.

- Provide opportunities for partners to *work together* on meaningful issues, and actively promote teamwork principles. Side issues or past conflicts should not prevent forward movement on the core issues facing the partnership today.

- Actively promote mutual understanding of the *short-term needs* and interests of all partners. People will not see the long term if certain immediate short-term needs are not met.

- Maintain a *balance* between short-term and long-term needs of all partners.

- Foster *leadership skills* among all partners; partners should be committed to the recruitment and retention of those with such skills.

- Identify *specific barriers* to the partnership; all concerned members should work together to eliminate them.

- Recognize the potential for *new structures* and *multiple structures* in order to support the needs and interests of all parties.

- *Evaluate and monitor* which models appear to work best, and spread the lessons learned to other relationships. This will require developing explicit objectives and performance measures for the relationship.

Experience suggests that the way to get to the more integrated models is by offering multiple models and approaches to physicians and actively managing all of them. Emerging evidence suggests that the more-integrated models are associated with physicians having more favorable attitudes toward the system regarding satisfaction, trust, loyalty, teamwork, collegiality, and related characteristics (Alexander and others, 1995).

Group Practice Formation

Little can be done to promote physician-system integration when most physicians are still practicing solo or in small partnerships. Thus, systems are using multiple approaches and strategies (as discussed above) to organize physicians into groups and to combine smaller groups into larger groups. Expanding practice management support services, providing start-up development funds, and visiting other sites were additional strategies used by the systems to expand physician participation in groups. All groups, of course, are not alike; they vary in size, specialty mix, method of compensation, management, governance, and related attributes. We believe the probability of practicing cost-effective medicine is greatest for multispecialty groups operating under full-risk contracts combined with incentive payment. The incentive payment should attempt to balance both productivity (number of patients seen) and quality (for example, patient satisfaction and functional health status measures) through use of an outcome management information system (Ellwood, 1988) that tracks patients and providers across the continuum of care. There is some evidence that physicians practicing in such groups experience stronger feelings of integration with the system than do physicians affiliated with the system through solo and small partnership practices (Schultz, Napiewocki, and Nerenz, 1994). Whether or not such practices are actually associated with more cost-effective care requires further study.

Perhaps the most important feature of group practice is the one least discussed. This is the ability to transfer knowledge and learning among individuals and different units of a system. To reduce the fragmentation that currently exists in the delivery of care and to replace it with more holistic practices will require a significant increase in the ability of health care organizations to transfer learning and knowledge from one part to another. It is much easier to communicate with five or six groups of physicians within a system than it is with three or four hundred separate physicians. It is much easier to develop protocols and pathways and to track outcomes and to learn from each other about best practices when physicians work together. It is also easier for physicians to manage and govern themselves in groups than it is to do so as relatively freestanding entities. This of course does not mean that groups will not disagree or have conflicting objectives, but they at least will have established management and governance mechanisms with which to address such challenges. The importance of group practice is, perhaps, best expressed by the words of one physician: "If you live in a world of eight-hundred-pound gorillas, it is better to be one than to have one sit on you."

Fairview's approach to aggregating physicians into group-like structures and attempting to speed up the transfer of knowledge and learning is discussed at the end of this chapter.

Infrastructure Support

The final key success factor for promoting physician-system integration involves administrative infrastructure support systems. While one can argue that all functional support processes such as finance, human resources, planning, and marketing are important, we found that two stood out: information systems and the use of CQI/TQM.

The study findings revealed that information systems were perceived to be among the least integrated functions within systems (Gillies and others, 1993), with as few as 11 percent of operating units sharing even a common patient identification number (Devers and others, 1994). It was therefore no surprise that the study systems were investing a significant amount of capital (as high as $150 million over three years in one case) in information systems. Most of this investment was going into developing a clinical/patient care data base that could link providers and patients across the continuum of care. Systems were learning that the initial challenge is not in automating the medical record (that is, creating the electronic medical record) but in figuring out what information is needed by what providers at what point in time across various delivery sites throughout the continuum. The information systems must serve multiple objectives, including providing aggregate data on cost, quality, and outcomes for after-the-fact analysis and reporting to external groups, as well as real-time information on patient clinical status and treatment plans from which immediate corrective action or changes in patient treatment can take place. In the process, the needs of different caregivers must be recognized. For example, primary care physicians and specialists will have different needs as will nurses, social workers, pharmacists, and other caregivers. Certain core information must therefore be available to all caregivers; in addition, there must be flexible modules that can be "called up" as needed to meet the specific needs of different caregivers. Only after these kinds of considerations are addressed does it make sense to consider automating the care record.

The number of health care organizations applying CQI/TQM has grown significantly over the past eight years. For example, 69 percent of hospitals report using CQI/TQM, with a significant percentage of these having done so within the last couple of years (Barsness and others, 1993). All of the study systems were active in implementing CQI/TQM processes, and two—Advocate and Henry Ford—won national awards for their efforts. While the systems were only beginning to document actual cost savings or better patient outcomes, each system believed that CQI/TQM was playing an essential role in promoting and facilitating physician-system and clinical integration.

There are many reasons for this. First, the philosophy of continuous improvement of quality resonates with health care professionals. Who can be against it? Second, the development of specific skills in identifying and dealing with variations from desired performance (for example, cause-and-effect diagrams, runs charts, Pareto charts, statistical process control charts, and so forth) provides everyone with a common tool kit and "language" for dealing with problems and opportunities for improvement. Third, the emphasis on empowerment and teamwork provides a shared culture that people across the system can buy into. Finally, the emphasis on fact-based, data-driven, results-based management appeals to physicians and other professionals trained as applied scientists. As will be further elaborated in Chapter Six, CQI/TQM practices and tools were the most prevalent methodology used by most systems in analyzing care processes, developing protocols, pathways, and case management systems, and examining data on the outcomes of these new approaches to patient treatment.

It is important to note that the effectiveness of most system CQI/TQM efforts was directly linked to three factors: (1) ongoing leadership and commitment from key individuals throughout the organization, (2) strong information systems that could support the effort, and (3) effective physician involvement. As one might expect, these three factors were themselves strongly intertwined such that if any one was missing, the other two were increasingly compromised.

Lack of physician involvement in CQI/TQM efforts was a particular problem for many systems. In most cases, physicians were not actually opposed to CQI/TQM but rather viewed it as "something the hospital was doing." This was often reinforced when hospitals, in fact, largely focused their efforts on such nonclinical processes as dietary, housekeeping, scheduling, billing, and related functions. In a couple of systems, however, there was more active opposition because the system's CQI/TQM efforts were framed primarily as cost-cutting approaches and were accompanied by staff layoffs. In these systems, physicians had an active distrust of CQI/TQM. These special issues aside, a common barrier faced by all systems was the lack of time physicians had available to actively participate in quality improvement efforts—even when physicians were most committed and when the process was focused on clinical issues.

Based on observation of the study systems and related research (Shortell, O'Brien, and others, 1995a; O'Brien, Shortell, and others, 1995; Blumenthal and Scheck, 1995), systems made the most progress when they focused their efforts on core clinical processes of importance to physicians; carefully segmented physicians into different groups in order to most fruitfully involve them in CQI/TQM efforts; and invested in clinical effectiveness and outcome support units, employing staff with statistical and data analysis skills to assist in designing, executing, and evaluating quality improvement efforts.

Among the most common clinical conditions addressed were acute myocardial infarction, coronary bypass graft surgery, stroke, pneumonia, C-section, chronic obstructive pulmonary disease, total hip replacement, asthma, and diabetes.

In regard to segmenting, it is useful to divide physicians into four groups: (1) natural enthusiasts, (2) salaried physicians, (3) physicians dealing with high-cost/high-volume conditions, and (4) the "neutral majority." Every system had a few physicians who were "turned on" by CQI approaches to practicing medicine. The strategy for these natural enthusiasts is a simple one of actively supporting and encouraging their enthusiasm. The second group, salaried physicians, is relatively easy to work with because they tend to be more organizationally committed to the system. For them, it is important to use quality improvement objectives and participation in continuous improvement efforts as part of their performance appraisal and incentive pay. Those physicians dealing with high-cost and/or high-volume conditions might receive special targeted educational efforts directly focused on conditions of clinical interest. Physicians in the first two groups can be used as peer leaders in assisting with this effort. Finally, those physicians constituting "the neutral majority" (which may be as high as 80 percent) should be approached with "just-in-time" training as specific issues of interest to them arise. Again, physicians in the first three groups can be used as peers in approaching the neutral majority. The important point is to recognize that not all physicians need to be involved equally or at the same time with CQI and to recognize that different approaches may be effective with different groups. Overall, information systems and CQI/TQM approaches go hand in hand as core infrastructure building blocks for physician alignment with health care systems.

Fairview Hospital and Healthcare Services

The home of Fairview Hospital and Healthcare Services (Fairview)—the twin cities of Minneapolis and St. Paul—is frequently described as one of the true examples of a "managed competition" health care market. While the Twin Cities are often cited for the development and consolidation of managed care companies, physician group practices, and hospital systems, until the early 1990s there had been little pressure to force the integration of all three players into organized delivery systems. The situation changed, however, when two watershed events created a substantial "zone of discomfort" for providers and managed care companies alike.

The first warning shot came from the employer community, specifically a group of fourteen of the Twin Cities' largest employers who collectively determined that the health care delivery system needed much more than a tune-up. This employer coalition took the form of the Business Health Care Action Group (BHCAG) and set out to accomplish "a fundamental restructuring of the local health care system via contractual performance requirements that support the provision of high quality, appropriate care in a coordinated, cost-effective manner." Further, the BHCAG had an expectation that the new system would be "a primary care based structure promoting high quality, necessary care [and would] demonstrate superior outcomes and continuous improvement over time."

The BHCAG sought to work selectively and as directly as possible with a limited provider panel to design a health care delivery system for members' 125,000 covered lives (employees, their families, and retirees). While the BHCAG was not able to contract directly with a provider group, the Group Care Consortium it selected (Group Health, MedCenters Health Plan, and the Mayo Clinic) was dominated by large multispecialty group practices with a substantial primary care presence. Neither Fairview nor the competing hospital-dominated health care systems—HealthSpan (now Allina), Health-East, and the University of Minnesota—were selected.

For the physicians on the medical staffs of Fairview's three Twin Cities hospitals, the limitations of the IPA with which it responded to the BHCAG's request for a proposal were apparent. The looseness of the structure, its inability to meaningfully implement and pursue quality improvement strategies, and the lack of an overarching integration strategy among the physicians and between physicians and Fairview all underscored the need for substantive change.

The second shot was fired from the public sector when a bipartisan leadership group in the Minnesota legislature created far-reaching health reform legislation. The most significant cost-containment and organizational changes outlined in the Minnesota Care bill called for health care to be purchased through integrated service networks (ISNs). The early definition of ISNs indicated that they were to be "organizations accountable for the costs and outcomes associated with delivering a full continuum of services to a defined population." The legislature had recognized the need to reform a "fragmented non-system of independent providers," many of whom were paid on a piecemeal basis, "into coordinated networks capable of providing all care for a fixed price."

Fairview had positioned itself in the Twin Cities through ownership in a joint venture preferred provider organization and a pluralistic approach to working with the physician community to pursue physician-system integration. Nevertheless, the two environmental shifts described above were enough to elicit considerable heartburn for Fairview's physicians and administrative ranks. As one physician in our study described it, "I understand that shifts happen, but this is a case of the shifts all hitting the fan at once, and you know what can happen in that scenario."

Physician-System Integration at Fairview Today

The discomfort zone created by the private and public sectors in the Twin Cities led to a monumental organizational planning process. A select group of physician leaders met weekly for several months to design a systemwide integrated practice network that today is referred to as Fairview Physicians Associates (FPA). FPA is a network of 645 physicians "who are affiliated to function and contract as a large, multi-specialty group and whose goal is to improve the quality and cost of care delivered to patients."

The Fairview Physicians Associates board of director structure is as follows:

- Six FPA member physicians (four primary care and two specialty care)
- Eight community members
- FPA president
- CEO of Fairview
- Clinic administrator representative

FPA's mission statement and organizational structure (Figure 5.2) appear below.

> FPA works with Fairview to advance the health of the community by continuously improving the quality of health care services delivered to individuals.
>
> FPA provides patients with access to personalized care through its network of small-to-medium-sized primary care and specialty clinics. These clinics share common support systems, patient care methodologies and aligned incentives in order to be accountable for delivering coordinated, cost-effective patient care.
>
> FPA's success is measured by improvements in the health outcomes of the individuals we serve, enhancements to the quality of the physician/patient relationship and the continued vitality of the network's practices.

As a physician-system organization, FPA has successfully developed relationships with three major managed care organizations, including the health plan sponsored by the Allina Health Systems—a major competitor of the Fairview system. A network-wide information system will be implemented in the near future, and a compensation methodology has been developed that rewards both productivity and performance.

Barriers and Challenges to Forming and Implementing FPA

FPA engaged in many of the same "meaningful discussions" held among primary care physicians and specialists and between physicians and hospitals throughout the country as they have pursued

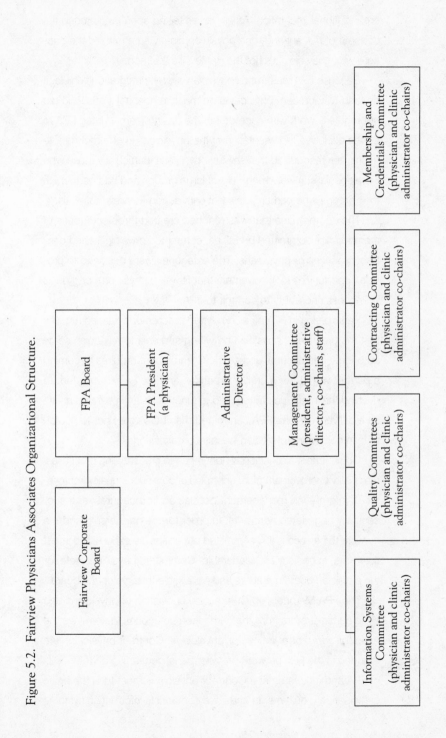

Figure 5.2. Fairview Physicians Associates Organizational Structure.

organizational integration. As all parties talked about and around the concept of risk sharing, one physician clearly summarized the concern when he said, "It's not the money, it's the money."

Because FPA was truly a physician-*system* integration vehicle, it needed to represent physicians on multiple hospital staffs who did not regularly work with each other. The design team wanted FPA to be the exclusive representative of the physicians in contract negotiations, but recognized that several physicians (particularly those who were specialists) were members of large groups and had partners in their groups who primarily saw patients at non-Fairview hospitals.

The compromise that was reached created three categories of membership: committed practices, committed physicians, and contract practices or physicians. The categories were designed to provide opportunities for involvement that fit with a physician's or group's willingness and ability to commit to FPA.

Participation in FPA as a *committed* practice or physician requires that the practice or physician be willing and able to relinquish some autonomy and assume some risk. Commitment requires becoming a partner with other member practices and the Fairview system to develop the infrastructure required to function as an integrated health care delivery system. FPA committed members agree not to participate in competing physician-hospital organizations.

Commitment also includes adherence to credentialing processes, the quality improvement plan, principles of continuous quality improvement, information management policies and procedures, and successfully negotiated contracts. In order for the partnership and the network to be successful, committed physicians are expected to invest their time, expertise, and leadership. Committed physicians vote for the physician board members and are eligible to serve on the board.

The FPA Membership Committee, consisting of physicians and clinic administrators from the committed categories, determines the need for *contract* practices or physicians. Contract physicians are included in the FPA network provider panel depending on the needs of FPA and its customers. Contract physicians must fulfill the basic participation requirements and have compatible information systems in place. Given the less comprehensive participation requirements and their freedom to be involved in competing physician-hospital organizations, contract physicians are not eligible to vote for physician board members or to serve on the board. Contract physicians may be asked to serve on quality improvement teams and to participate in clinical pathway development activities.

Where is Fairview Headed?

Fairview as a system has firmly decided that FPA will be the physician organization with which it partners in managed care contracting and integrated delivery system development. Although Fairview has been active in the acquisition of primary care practices, the employed physicians are represented by FPA and will continue to be so represented in the future.

The organization that fired the first warning shot of private sector health reform—the BHCAG—has now grown to represent nearly 250,000 covered lives and has announced plans to renegotiate its exclusive relationship to include other primary care–based organizations like FPA. Representatives for both BHCAG and FPA characterize what FPA has done as a good fit for BHCAG.

As FPA goes forward, it is implementing a unique *fee-for-quality* compensation methodology for its members, whereby physicians will be paid more or less depending on how well they perform relative to key performance measures developed by the FPA Contracting and Product Development Committee. The incentive is not to do less just because the organization as a whole may be capitated. Rather, the incentive is to have the right intervention, delivered at the right time, in the right place, with the right result. As these standards evolve, physicians who follow the standards (protocols, pathways, and so on) will be compensated better than those who do not.

Sharp HealthCare

Sharp HealthCare, based in San Diego, California, is the largest not-for-profit health care corporation in San Diego. Sharp has progressed in many areas important to physician integration, yet it continues to face the growing pains of a newly developed system: 33 percent of Sharp's operating units have been added since 1989. In addition, 67 percent of Sharp's operating units have joined the system through merger or acquisition. This growth has understandably presented challenges to Sharp's physician integration efforts.

Progress Toward Physician Integration

By 1990, Sharp was well along in the development of its integrated delivery network. A key event was the acquisition of Rees-Stealy as a staff-model multispecialty group practice in 1985. Currently, Sharp Rees-Stealy medical group operates at 90 percent capitation. To ensure that the system remained adaptable during the early stages of development, all programs and facilities were designed with the understanding that flexibility would be critical to survival. Likewise, Sharp began developing systemwide information systems in the early stages of growth.

Early in the development of the Sharp system, participants reported concerns of trying to "hit a moving target," an indication of inconsistent goals and incentives. Schisms arose not only between the most recently added physicians and hospitals and those of more significant tenure with Sharp, but also between the hospitals and the physicians in general. Sharp's primary challenge was to understand these different groups and create common incentives that would serve the system as a whole. In concert with the aligning of goals and incentives, Sharp has recognized the necessity of thorough communication and education of all participants.

Common Incentives

Since its inception, Sharp has sought to create a common vision designed to permeate the entire system; thus management philosophy maintains both a centralized focus and a decentralized focus. For instance, within Sharp's corporate management, there are incentives for the success of specific operating units as well as for the system overall, conveying the importance of individual performance for the betterment of the Sharp system.

In addition, Sharp has restructured its operations such that hospitals (and their medical staffs) and physician groups are organized separately. While this may serve them well in some areas in the short term, ultimately problems may arise due to the divergent interests and incentives of the hospitals and the medical groups. In particular, some sources indicate that there may be more competition than cooperation between some physician groups and hospitals. Moreover, this may accentuate fear and distrust on the part of physicians, leading to barriers to development between these two entities.

Internal Factors: Managing Fear and Distrust

Because many pieces of Sharp's network are newly formed, fear and distrust on the part of staff and physicians present a wide variety of challenges for Sharp's integration efforts. Many staff concerns must be resolved quickly, and lines of communication must remain open both to and from the corporate office. In resolving cultural dilemmas arising from mergers as well as from rapid growth and development, Sharp has learned the benefits of staff empowerment.

To further prepare for managed care, Sharp has developed a utilization management function that operates under the physician practice area rather than under the hospital. The success of this decision will depend on the extent to which the physicians have a broad view of utilization management that encompasses both cost containment and quality initiatives. Any dissension caused by this arrangement may be compounded by newly added hospitals and physician groups that may not understand current goals and incentives. Thus the system's overall objectives must be conveyed to all involved in order to create the most beneficial environment for appropriate utilization review. Current results from Sharp reveal quantifiable improvement and positive feedback from those involved with this effort, but long-term results will determine the true success of this program.

Interviews with Sharp respondents revealed that change remains an important core value throughout the organization. Moreover, these groups reported operating under a philosophy that recognizes the increasing roles of creativity and innovation. This systemwide belief will serve Sharp well as it faces the emerging challenges of integrating physicians and systems of care.

Primary Care Physicians Versus Specialists

Sharp follows the current belief that primary care physicians should serve as the entry point to the system, and in support of this belief Sharp has established a family practice residency program. Across all structures of the Sharp system, integration efforts focus on cost and quality, attempting to benefit from primary care physicians as a cost-effective entry point for patient care. Although system administration has sought the input of primary care physicians in its development of strategies, some primary care physicians have been slow to understand their role in the system environment as they now manage the care of a large population of patients. This lack of understanding has increased the importance of physician education as well as communication between administration and physician groups.

Sharp currently estimates that its primary care/specialist ratio is still skewed toward specialists, who make up about 60 percent of the physicians. Sharp has begun retraining internists and other specialists in order to increase the number of practicing primary care physicians; it also makes extensive use of physician assistants and nurse practitioners.

Physician Leadership Development

Sharp recognizes that teams will play a crucial role in its integration efforts. In order to move these teams toward common system goals, Sharp must spark the interest of physician leaders across the system. Without the power of physician leaders within specific groups or institutions, Sharp will have little success in motivating change. Sharp must continue to take advantage of physician leaders by placing them in the corporate office; an example of this practice, not atypical within the Sharp system, is that the leaders of Sharp Memorial Hospital currently include both a physician and a nurse.

Sharp has made a variety of efforts to enhance physician integration through education and leadership development. Included in these efforts is the Managed Care Forum, which operates with the following goal in mind: "The forum was designed to afford those groups committed to Sharp and managed care an opportunity to come together in a collaborative manner for the sharing of common resources and expertise."

The Managed Care Forum has allowed individuals involved with Sharp to better understand the managed care environment. For physicians, this forum has provided an opportunity to recognize the impact of managed care on the entire system. Armed with this understanding, physicians are now better prepared to modify their behavior to the benefit of the overall system. To further encourage team building and system thinking among physicians, Sharp has altered its medical training to include sections that socialize physicians to the new practice environment.

In addition to physician leadership development, Sharp has also trained its staff in leadership skills. This movement has been motivated by the understanding that while physicians are critical to the changing health care arena, all staff members must participate in new process development. In an attempt to ensure that all participants are motivated to work for the betterment of the overall system, Sharp has strived for empowerment throughout each level of the organization. Sharp's recognition that empowerment is fundamental to successful change and quality improvement has driven much of its integration success.

Implementation of Integrated Information Systems

As Sharp consolidates its various operating units and physician groups, integrated information systems (IS) will prove critical. Sharp is currently working to develop an electronic medical record, but a full-scale application is not yet available. As this technology comes on-line, Sharp will begin to benefit from the abundance of information it maintains through its integrated system. By 1996, Sharp will have invested $30 million to create a new information system that centralizes clinical and financial resources. In order to fully capitalize on the integrated system, Sharp must continue to focus efforts on developing IS technology. This IS development ultimately will allow all participants to communicate more efficiently, improving the timeliness and quality of information generated systemwide. More important, it will enable all participants to work from the same information set, significantly improving physician understanding of the rapidly changing environment in which they practice and thus improving physician integration.

Sharp's efforts are focused on the goal of developing a common system; in fact, this is a "condition of affiliation." By carefully monitoring their information system development, many of Sharp's affiliates have ensured that their IS will be compatible with the overall system. As the aforementioned efforts improve overall system integration, Sharp will be capable of increased system development.

One must ask the critical questions of when these systems will be on-line and how much they will be altered to become functionally integrated. Likewise, Sharp must address the issue of educating system users accustomed to other IS formats. In the long term, Sharp will benefit from its IS development only if IS implementation is tied to Sharp's overall integration growth, linking incentives and processes across all groups.

Creating a Zone of Manageable Discomfort

The task of creating a zone of manageable discomfort has proven challenging for Sharp, yet progress is being made. This task can succeed only if continuous pressure is applied evenly and appropriately systemwide. With this in mind, one can understand the potential difficulties Sharp's leadership has as it motivates varied participants: what is too slow for one group may be too fast for another. Whereas some of the players have tested the waters of managed care, others have effectively avoided it and fear immediate immersion.

Maintaining the interest of diverse groups provides challenges for Sharp, but the value of the lessons it has learned will likely outweigh the problems. For instance, hospitals whose integration efforts are more fully developed may show by example what lies ahead. Likewise, physician groups that have become fully integrated with Sharp HealthCare can convey through their actions the benefits of integration. Models of success and best practices have been and will continue to be useful for the Sharp system.

Communicating the Vision

Sharp has proven very successful in determining long-term system vision; however, systemwide vision remains clouded for some of the noncorporate staff. This problem is exacerbated by the variation in internal organizational structures and cultures among physician groups and hospitals. To effectively address its competitors, Sharp must ensure that all within the organization work toward the same end goal on a systemwide level. To this end, Sharp recognizes the importance of initiating exchange among all groups. In an attempt to improve overall communication—and thus promote a common vision—Sharp has restructured such that administrators are responsible for specific divisions across the entire system. This change has improved system integration and improved systemwide communication by creating common incentives. Sharp's communication of direction relies heavily on its CEO, renowned within the organization as a visionary. Moreover, the CEO maintains the respect and trust of those below him, leading the vast majority to embrace his vision for growth and development.

Empowering Physicians

As Sharp has revised organizational structures, they have increased physician involvement, recognizing that several factors related to physician empowerment will determine the success of the integrated system. First, physicians inclined to improve operational status will promote change and defuse grass roots dissent. Moreover, by involving physicians in integration from the beginning and from the ground up, Sharp ensures that new systems are designed to benefit specific physicians, group practices, individual hospitals, and the system itself. With physicians leading clinical change, new systems will be created in the most efficient manner.

Pluralistic Approaches and Models

Sharp benefits from its pluralistic approach to working with physicians. Currently, the majority of physicians operate within the following structures: affiliated group practices or IPAs, foundations, MSOs, hospital medical staffs, and/or clinics, in which they are partners. This variety of approaches has allowed a large number of physicians to become directly affiliated with the Sharp system, thereby beginning much-needed business relationships. Increased variety allows Sharp to appeal to physicians who remain more cautious of widespread integration and the limitations they feel it may create.

For all the benefits pluralistic approaches to physician management create, some liabilities do exist. One of these involves how physicians will view those who have chosen alternative management structures. Will those who have chosen to work under staff models resent those who have remained in independent practices, and will the latter feel that the former are creating dead weight?

Group Practice Formation

In assessing the maturity of Sharp's group practice development, several challenges come to the fore, one of which is the strength of Sharp's individual medical groups. Without question, the power they maintain separately could deter integration as they strive to maintain individuality. On the other hand, counter to concerns of maladjusted autonomy, Sharp's efforts to form group practices benefit from the pluralistic approaches Sharp offers physicians. As the physicians maintain some autonomy and flexibility in practice structure, it becomes more likely that they will embrace the system and cooperate with integration objectives. As noted earlier, preliminary research reveals that these autonomous systems can integrate effectively with the proper incentive structures; the challenge will be to align all incentives and operations across these groups of physicians.Sharp's initial efforts in group practice remain successful, but long-term integration hinges on how these varied groups are included in system redesign. Key to this will be the extent to which Sharp can secure sufficient capital to create equity relationships with its physicians.

Key Success Factors

Sharp's quality assurance and improvement efforts have proven successful and will benefit Sharp in the long term. Sharp has created an environment in which quality is first assessed and improved at the local level and then shared at the system level. Thus, those closest to the original problem create solutions and inform others of this potentially beneficial information, ensuring appropriate implementation as well as reduced loss of information for the system. Sharp must now leverage its experience with coalition and empowerment to further its physician integration objectives.

Whereas many quality efforts evolve from individual units, case management and care paths are generally instituted on a systemwide scale, usually because of the significant financial resources required to make changes in this area. This conflict of system versus local direction often detracts from protocol development and implementation, thereby significantly reducing the probability of success. As physician integration improves, with physicians and staff defining their efforts on a system level, protocols may be more readily developed and embraced. Likewise, the protocols, if managed appropriately, should serve as a unifying operative for all participants, further benefiting physician integration efforts.

As discussed earlier, empowerment has proven integral to the successful integration of the Sharp system. Likewise, by educating all participants and encouraging open communication throughout the organization, Sharp has increased its staff members' understanding of the changing health care marketplace. Sharp benefits from their educated responses as they react more appropriately to the alterations taking place than they would in the face of an unknown threat.

Sharp's Future Challenges

As Sharp looks to the future, it must consider a myriad of issues. Securing sufficient capital to explore long-run equity relationships with its physicians is critical. Sharp's current efforts to create a 50/50 joint venture with Columbia/HCA may be a significant step in this direction. With rapid growth and development and an increasingly diversified collection of participants, Sharp may have difficulty maintaining perspective for the entire system; it must continue to focus on clearly defining its systemwide strategy. As Sharp further diversifies into insurance products, it must continue to readdress strategic goals as well as competitors' responses. As already discussed, although the system has made important strides in its integration efforts, achieving long-lasting partnerships with relatively diverse groups of physicians is likely to be an ongoing challenge.

Future Issues

As organized delivery systems evolve, they will face three major issues in their effort to build increasing physician-system integration. These involve accepting increased risk for the health of the populations they serve; working out accountability and control issues within the partnership; and broadening the continuum of care.

To the extent that health care is paid for on a prepaid capitated or similar basis, systems—having earned their revenue up front—assume major responsibility for the health of those covered. As a result, selectivity issues arise in terms of managing adverse risk—in other words, how will the system handle individuals with poor health status who are likely to be disproportionate users of services? While the adverse risk problem may be dealt with to some extent through risk-adjusted payments, stop-loss coverage, and/or reinsurance, it is also likely that some residual responsibility will be borne by providers. Because of this, there are incentives for more cost-effective management of chronic and end-stage illnesses and of high-risk individuals in general. This will require high degrees of coordination and collaboration among physicians, nurses, other caregivers, and the multiple settings in which such care is provided. This, in turn, may result in greater use of staff and equity models of physician organization (Cave, 1995). Most study systems were exploring ways of more closely aligning physician and system economic interests for the long run using equity or similar arrangements. In many cases, this will likely require additional infusions of capital and a search for partners who share similar values and interests.

In addition to the responsibility for enrolled lives, many systems will also become involved in maintaining the health of the entire geographic population they serve. This is particularly true for systems located in urban areas with higher proportions of uninsured and medically indigent individuals and for systems whose mission emphasizes serving the poor and needy. These systems will become increasingly involved in disease prevention and health promotion activities such as immunizations, prenatal care, health education, and management of domestic violence. In so doing, these systems will work jointly with other health care organizations, public health departments, social service agencies, schools, and related community groups. They will do so not only because they believe it is the "right thing to do" but also because it makes economic sense. It is less costly to immunize a child against measles than it is to treat the aftereffects; providing prenatal care that leads to a healthy birth is more cost-effective than providing neonatal intensive care (Washington State Health Care Commission, 1992). Systems such as Advocate, Fairview, Franciscan, Henry Ford, and Sisters of Providence are finding that dealing with these issues requires an increased permeability of boundaries between the health care delivery system and other organizations in the community. It requires physicians and other health care professionals to extend their notion of coordinated care beyond the formal boundaries of the personal health care system and to become more involved in issues of crime, safety, domestic violence, education, housing, and the environment.

The second set of future issues revolves around accountability and control as the partnership between physicians and the delivery system matures. Accountability demands by multiple stakeholders will involve more explicit information on the cost, quality, and outcomes of care. These demands will require more interdependent, collaborative, and cooperative behavior on the part of physicians, other caregivers, and health care executives to produce such data and to withstand the increased scrutiny. At the same time, control issues will be a continuing challenge. Physicians, understandably, want to continue to control their professional destiny but will need to do so in increasingly interdependent and complex relationships with others. As suggested in this chapter, this will require many physicians to assume more responsible managerial and governance roles within the system, and to work collaboratively with health care executives and with other health care professionals in teams. Issues of how to most equitably divide revenue payments—between primary care physicians and specialists, between and among medical groups, and between physicians and the hospitals—will assume increased importance. The challenges of how best to treat patients and incorporate new medical technologies will involve not only potential conflicts among physicians but also between physicians and other members of the health care team. These issues are not new, of course, but will be accentuated by the new demands for more cost-effective care and a structurally reorganized health care system. Those systems and physicians that continuously work on their relationship will be the best able to deal with these issues. They will embrace the "six I's" of effective strategic partnership found in other settings: importance, investment, interdependence, integrated, informed, and institutionalized (Kanter, 1989). They will work to ensure that the relationship remains strategically *impor-*

tant to all parties. The focus will be on maintaining and increasing "covered lives" tied together by shared economic incentives. They will look at the relationship as a long-term *investment,* with rewards balancing out over the long run as evidenced by the growth of salaried and equity models. Most important, they will look for opportunities to increase their *interdependence,* because the marketplace and other external forces will demand it. Most physicians do not have the capital or the managerial and organizational expertise to go it entirely alone. Hospitals and other health care organizations, on the other hand, do not and cannot practice medicine. Thus, there is an almost inherent tendency toward interdependence. As suggested by this chapter, these interdependent relationships will become increasingly *integrated* through the further development of group practice, more sophisticated information systems, and greater physician involvement in management and governance of the system. As a result, the relationship will become more *informed,* as all parties are involved in joint strategic planning, implementation, monitoring, and evaluation. Finally, as the relationship becomes more interdependent, integrated, and informed, it also becomes more *institutionalized* in terms of developing an infrastructure of trust. Although cracks in the relationship will inevitably develop, the more mature partnerships will have a reservoir of past relationships, past performance, past success, informed data bases, and a positive culture that enables the cracks to be repaired.

The final challenge to physicians in systems will be to continue to build an integrated continuum of care from primary care, to acute care, to restorative care, to maintenance care. This involves both breadth and depth of care, and the capital required to ensure both. There is need to have sufficient breadth of services across a given geographic area—particularly in regard to disease prevention, health promotion, and primary care. There is also need for some degree of depth—having more than one site offer the service within the system—in order to deal with demand as well as geographic coverage. New technologies and treatment practices, the results of clinical reengineering, and consumer preferences will also affect the number, type, and configuration of services across the continuum. In facing these issues, physicians may come to realize that their best chance for maintaining some degree of autonomy, influence, and sense of professional identity will, in essence, lie in being willing to establish cooperative relationships with health care systems.

. . . .

Clinical Integration
Maximizing Patient Value

*Clinical integration is like pornography. Everyone
recognizes it when they see it.*

The quotation above from a study respondent suggests that clinical integration is an umbrella concept reflecting many specific meanings and interpretations. Among these are the notions of continuity of care, coordination of care, disease stage management, good communication among caregivers, smooth transfer of information and records, elimination of duplicate testing and procedures, and, in general, making sure that things don't "fall between the cracks." We have previously defined clinical integration as the extent to which patient care services are coordinated across people, functions, activities, and sites so as to maximize the value of services delivered to patients. We believe it is the most important element in the ability of organized delivery systems to achieve more cost-effective delivery of care because it is most directly associated with the direct provision of such care. The issue is well stated as follows:

> In the perfect world of a fully integrated medical
> system, each clinical decision—whether it be a decision regarding drug therapy versus surgery, ambulatory
> care versus hospital admission, or nutritional counselling versus psychological counselling—would be

determined by answering the question: "How can we the providers and the system restore the patient's health using the smallest amount of total resources?" In the real world, imperfect information, incomplete communication, conflicting incentives, and organizational/professional biases hinder providers' ability to ask as well as answer that question. An integrated system's goal is to create organizational structures, provide technical support, and offer positive and negative sanctions that counteract those influences. [Institute for the Future, 1993a]

Many of the challenges to clinical integration are associated with the problems of achieving functional and physician-system integration; however, clinical integration also faces its own unique challenges, which are highlighted in this chapter. We also present some key results related to clinical integration and some of the factors associated with more successful efforts. We then discuss some of the future challenges.

Primary Findings

The following sections describe the degree of clinical integration among the study systems and the key relationships among the factors involved. Findings are presented at both the system and individual hospital levels.

Degree of Integration

Table 6.1 summarizes some of the more important findings regarding objective measures of clinical integration.

What is most striking is the relative lack of progress between 1991 and 1992 on most measures. The major exceptions are in regard to the number of clinical protocols developed (although the percentage actually shared with other units declined) and the increase in clinical outcome data collection and sharing among the units. In other areas such as medical records' uniformity and accessibility, shared clinical support services, shared clinical service lines, and clinical programming and planning efforts, there was relatively little or no change other than that more operating units shared a physician recruitment plan.

The lack of progress is not surprising. Clinical integration is extremely difficult work, and one year is far too short a period to discern measurable progress in most areas. The active use of clinical outcome data is encouraging. For example, nearly all operating units were using at least some outcome measures—80 percent for continuous improvement purposes, 75 percent for physician credentialing efforts, and 52 percent for purposes of HMO contracting. Nonetheless, the system respondents themselves scored their clinical integration efforts a 2.5 (on a 1-to-5 low-to-high scale) in both 1991 and 1992. In 1994, the mean assessment was only 2.4. Below, we briefly highlight those variables that were most significantly associated with clinical integration.

Key Relationships

Among the key findings regarding clinical integration were the following:

- Systems that developed more internally than through merger and acquisition were *less* clinically integrated.

- Functional integration was generally not related to the objective measures of clinical integration.

- Depth of services offered was positively associated with clinical integration.

- Standardization was positively associated with clinical integration. In particular, the standardization of information systems was positively associated as expected with the degree and uniformity of medical records sharing, which in turn was positively associated with shared

Table 6.1. Objective Measures of Clinical Integration.

Concept or measure	Fiscal year 1991 $\overline{X}$ (Standard deviation; Range)	Fiscal year 1992 $\overline{X}$ (Standard deviation; Range)
Clinical protocol development		
number of protocols per operating unit	2.9[a] (5; 0–16)	14.1 (22; 0–70)
percent protocols shared with at least one other operating unit	61.5 (32; 25–100)	32.5 (42; 0–100)
Medical records uniformity and accessibility		
percent medical records features shared	10.9 (15; 0–48)	13.5 (15; 0–46)
percent patient identification features shared	11.4 (18; 0–44)	9.6 (13; 0–33)
percent operating units (OUs) with electronic access to at least one other OU	9.5 (17; 0–43)	7.8 (12; 0–27)
percent OUs with electronic access within the OU	38.5 (46; 0–100)	34.0 (38; 0–100)
percent OUs using an integrated record with problem-oriented flow sheet	5.0 (17; 0–55)	10.0 (19; 0–50)

Clinical outcomes data collection		
number of 15 clinical outcomes collected only	5.3[a] (9; 0–12)	8.6 (4; 2–15)
number of 15 clinical outcomes collected and shared	1.9 (3; 0–9)	3.4 (3; 0–9)
Clinical programming and planning efforts		
percent OUs sharing a PHO	12.8 (30; 0–100)	15.2 (29; 0–90)
percent OUs sharing a recruitment plan	42.3 (47; 0–100)	65.1 (34; 0–100)
Shared clinical support services		
number of 9 support services shared	1.4 (1; 0–4)	1.6 (2; 0–5)
Shared clinical service lines		
number of 10 clinical service lines shared with at least one other OU	1.27 (1.7; 0–5.1)	1.26 (1.3; 0–4.1)
System integration	FY 1991	FY 1992 FY 1994
perceived clinical integration	2.5 (.3; 2–3)	2.5 (.2; 2–3) 2.4 (.2; 2–3)

[a]Significantly different at .05 one tailed

clinical service lines (for example, cardiovascular, oncology, behavioral medicine) and shared clinical support services (for example, lab, pharmacy, radiology).

- Physician-system integration was strongly and consistently associated with clinical integration, as predicted. The relationships were particularly strong for the group practice measures. Also, the greater the percentage of physicians in management positions with responsibilities *across* two or more institutions, the greater the degree of common medical staff organization structure and shared credentialing.

- There was generally no relationship between clinical integration and financial performance. This is not surprising given the low levels of clinical integration occurring within the study systems at the time.

Analysis at the individual hospital level revealed several findings of interest. First, larger hospitals (as measured by beds) are more likely to share clinical protocols, clinical outcome measures, and medical records. Second, the greater the distance between hospitals, the less likely they are to share clinical service lines or support services such as lab, radiology, and pharmacy. Third, hospitals that were owned by a system from the beginning were less likely to share clinical service lines or clinical support services. Fourth, the greater the percentage of physicians practicing in groups and, in particular, in groups of twenty-five or more, the more likely were their associated hospitals to share clinical service lines, clinical support services, and medical records. Fifth, the greater the degree of physician administrative involvement and common credentialing, the more likely the hospital was to share clinical service lines, clinical support services, medical records, clinical outcomes and protocols. Sixth, hospitals with a prospector strategic orientation were further along in their clinical integration efforts on almost all of the above measures. Seventh, a greater degree of HMO market penetration was associated with more shared clinical outcomes and shared medical records.

The above findings generally support the hypothesized relationships discussed in Chapter Three. As was the case for physician-system integration discussed in the preceding chapter, these findings provide an empirical foundation for discussion of the barriers and challenges as well as success factors highlighted in the following sections.

Barriers and Challenges

Clinical integration requires difficult, lifelong work. This is the most fundamental lesson from the study and is emphasized by others as well (for example, see Conrad, 1993). Unlike implementing an information system or recruiting a targeted number of primary care physicians, clinical integration is not something that one declares "finished" at a given point in time or after spending a fixed sum of resources or effort. It is an inherently difficult process because it involves reorganization of the medical profession and of relationships among physicians, nurses, and other health care professionals; reinvention of the American hospital; incorporation of new technologies and treatment practices; and ongoing adaptation to new payment arrangements and patient preferences. The challenge is to integrate across time, place, profession, and technology. These challenges will grow in importance as chronic illnesses loom larger.

Based on our field work and related research (O'Brien, Shortell, and others, 1995), we use four dimensions—the strategic, the structural, the cultural, and the technical—to understand the barriers to clinical integration. The *strategic* dimension emphasizes that clinical integration activities must focus on strategically important issues facing the system, not on peripheral activities. Clinical integration must focus on a sufficient breadth of activity to have real meaning for the system. The *structural* dimension refers to the overall organizational structure of the system to support clinical integration efforts. It also refers to task forces, committees, councils, work groups, and related arrangements for diffusing clinical integration efforts and "best practices" throughout the system. The *cultural* dimension refers to the underlying beliefs, values, norms, and behavior of the system, which either support or inhibit clinical integration. Finally, the *technical* dimension refers to the extent to which those associated with the system have the necessary training and skills to achieve clinical integration objectives. It also includes the extent to which an information system is in place to achieve such objectives.

In order to achieve high degrees of clinical integration, systems must attend to all four dimensions simultaneously and attempt to align them with each other. Table 6.2 shows what happens when one or another dimension is missing.

When the strategic dimension is missing, nothing really important gets done. Clinical integration efforts have relatively little impact because they are not focused on the strategic priorities of the system. When the structural component is missing, one observes pockets of clinical integration success but little organization-wide or systemwide impact. This is because the structures for diffusing the learning and best practices throughout the organization and system are absent. When the cultural component is missing, nothing lasts. Short-run successes fall apart because the organization lacks an overall culture that supports clinical integration. Absence of the technical dimension results in frustration and false starts. People do not have the necessary multiskilled training in TQM techniques necessary to support clinical integration activity. It is only when all four dimensions are worked on simultaneously and are aligned with each other that real progress occurs. This is, of course, a difficult challenge, one that makes achieving meaningful levels of clinical integration both an ongoing, lifelong process and a real source of potential sustainable competitive advantage.

Using the above framework, we found that the most significant barriers to clinical integration among the study systems were as follows: (1) lack of a specific strategy and implementation plan for

Table 6.2. Components Needed to Achieve Clinical Integration Across the Continuum of Care.

Strategic	Structural	Cultural	Technical	Result
0	1	1	1	No significant impact on anything really important
1	0	1	1	Inability to capture the learning and spread it throughout the organization
1	1	0	1	Small, temporary effects; no lasting impact
1	1	1	0	Frustration and false starts
1	1	1	1	Lasting systemwide impact

Note: 1 = Present; 0 = Absent

achieving clinical integration; (2) lack of or misalignment of internal incentives to achieve clinical integration; (3) too few physician groups; (4) dispersed geography; (5) the institutional autonomy of hospitals; (6) employee fears of job loss and physician fears of autonomy loss; (7) inadequate information systems; and (8) lack of population-based planning. At the outset, one must also recognize that clinical integration will not proceed very far without (1) economic pressures in the marketplace and/or public policy demanding it, (2) a regulatory and legal framework permitting various forms of consolidation and partnerships, and (3) personnel credentialing and licensing laws and practices that promote greater flexibility in the use of health personnel. These issues are discussed more fully in Chapter Eight.

Strategic Barriers

Although all systems aspired to become more integrated and saw clinical integration as central to such achievement, few had a specific plan to accomplish it. All systems made extensive use of strategic planning processes and practices, but most of the activities centered on cost reductions and on development of new services and products for purposes of managed care contracting. Although these plans would often include elements of clinical integration such as the intent to eliminate redundant services or to relocate such services, it was difficult to discern a coherent thread. In brief, there did not appear to be an overall plan for clinical integration itself within the context of the systems' overall strategic plan. Nor was anyone specifically charged with accountability for achieving clinical integration objectives in a concerted fashion. As a result, clinical integration activity largely occurred in fits and starts, with efforts in one area largely unrelated or unknown to those working in other areas. In many respects, the lack of a specific clinical integration plan reflected most systems' relative lack of awareness of the importance of clinical integration to achieving system goals. As previously noted, most systems had assembled the pieces of the continuum of care but were not very far advanced in bringing them together. Most systems were still working on the precursors to clinical integration: putting together a functional infrastructure and working on physician-system integration issues. During the course of the study, most systems' appreciation of the importance of clinical integration grew dramatically, and with this came an increased focus on developing specific plans and establishing accountability.

Structural Barriers

The study systems experienced three types of structural barriers: missing or misaligned incentives, too few physician groups, and dispersed geography.

Missing or Misaligned Incentives

Most systems had developed a few clinical service lines in such areas as cardiovascular, behavioral medicine, or cancer care. These service lines were typically organized around multidisciplinary teams from different functional areas charged with caring for patients across all settings. These changes in organization structure, however, were usually *not* accompanied by changes in budgeting, performance appraisal, and reward practices and policies. Physicians, nurses, and other health professionals were asked to work more collaboratively to provide greater continuity of care, but budgeting would often be based on meeting hospital department targets. Similarly, performance appraisal would be based on traditional criteria linked to inpatient settings, and rewards were based on accomplishment of individual goals and objectives rather than on group or team objectives. As a result, members of the multidisciplinary team often worked at cross-purposes, caught up in a web of conflicting incentives and motivations. For example, one nurse interviewed expressed her frustration with being unable to use training and education resources for her team's development because it would have caused the nursing department's budget to be overspent. Others complained that their annual employee performance review was still being conducted by the department head, who knew little about their performance on the cross-functional team. And many noted that their actual compensation still seemed to be largely individually based rather than group or team based. Thus, efforts to provide more integrated care were frustrated by budgeting and human resource practices and policies that were not only inconsistent but often in opposition to the effective function of multidisciplinary teams.

Too Few Physician Groups

Providing more integrated care requires high levels of communication, information transfer, learning, and trust in addition to competent technical skills. It is extremely difficult to achieve these levels when physicians are largely isolated from each other, practicing solo or in small partnerships or even in small group practices of three to six physicians. In such practices, there is little opportunity to learn from each other, to influence each other's behavior, to work on developing protocols and care management systems, or to collaborate with nurses and other health professionals in such undertakings. These issues become particularly problematic for patients with multiple illnesses or with chronic disease. For example, patients with advanced cancer have been known to see an average of three different physicians about fifteen times within a three-month period (Mor and Rice, 1993). Such a process places significant coordination and communication demands on the physicians as well as the patients, increasing the likelihood that treatment compliance will be compromised. This may be a particular problem for less well educated patients or where the physician and the patient speak different languages. Group practices, particularly multispecialty groups where physicians are in closer contact with each other, are likely to mitigate the adverse consequences of using so many different providers. In fact, group practices may *reduce* the number of providers that need to be seen in the first place.

Dispersed Geography

The greatest opportunities for clinical integration exist in local area networks and markets. This is because patients are only willing to travel so many miles for care, which in turn influences physician locational choices. Within these perimeters, physicians establish referral patterns and identify with local hospitals, which establishes boundaries for clinical integration opportunities. We measured the distances of all operating units from each other for a given system, and found that systems with a greater than fifty-mile average distance among its facilities had significantly lower scores on clinical integration. It is simply more difficult to establish shared clinical service lines, support services, personnel, and related aspects of clinical integration when facilities are widely dispersed across a geographic area. Recognizing the impact of geographic distance, a number of systems (for example, Advocate and Sutter) changed their structures, organizing into subregions more consistent with patient care-seeking preferences and physician practices and referral behavior.

Cultural Barriers

Our study identified two cultural barriers to clinical integration: the institutional autonomy of hospitals and the fears of employees and physicians.

Institutional Autonomy of Hospitals

A significant cultural constraint to clinical integration was the entrenched institutional autonomy of hospitals. With possibly one exception, all of the study systems had developed around hospitals as the hub of the system. In all cases, the systems' hospitals generated the most revenue for system growth and expansion. Thus, it was natural for hospitals, particularly those considered to be the flagship institution of the system, to think of themselves as the center. This attitude was, of course, reinforced by the hospitals' local boards of trustees. The result was that these hospitals would frequently block such clinical integration efforts as sharing laboratory services, relocating services to other areas of the system, or taking on new services and programs that they did not traditionally view as part of their mission (Shortell, Gillies, and others, 1993). Efforts to encourage cooperation between or among hospitals would often get bogged down over issues of who was going to "control" the service. In other cases, such as managed care contracting, cooperative efforts were undermined by differences in the cost structures of the individual hospitals: the lower-cost hospitals would not want to be part of a contract with a higher-cost hospital for fear of losing the contract. Evidence outside of the present study also highlights the difficulties involved. For example, a recent study of seventeen integrated delivery networks indicated that only 53 percent were even willing to consider consolidating accounting services, only 41 percent were willing to consider consolidating lab services, and only 18 percent were willing to consider consolidating cancer treatment, diagnostic imaging, orthopedics, or surgical services (Scott, 1995). It appears that much work remains to be done in order to create the "new American hospital" (Sherman, 1993).

Fears

The second major cultural barrier to clinical integration is fear. Hospital employees were fearful that efforts to form a more clinically integrated continuum of care would or could result in loss of their jobs. Physicians were afraid that clinical integration was a threat to the independence of their practices and the resources currently available to them. They were also concerned that cost and clinical outcome data would, in the words of one physician, "be used against us." These concerns and fears are legitimate and understandable but were particularly pronounced in those organizations with more hierarchical cultures and cultures emphasizing cost containment, as compared to those emphasizing teamwork and the relationships that would support risk taking in the search for creative solutions to problems.

Technical Barriers

Our study shows that the two main technical barriers to clinical integration were underdeveloped information systems and inadequate population-based planning.

Information Systems

As we found for physician-system integration, inadequate information systems represented a significant barrier to clinical integration. The challenge lies in developing the capability to track patients and providers across the continuum of care. Particularly important are the "handoff" stages, such as at admission to the hospital from the primary care physician's or specialist physician's office; hospital discharge to the next setting of care such as the nursing home, physician office, or home; and subsequent patient encounters that occur with different providers and/or treatment settings. Providers and patients alike were frequently frustrated by the lack of timely or accurate information; redundant questions and the rescheduling of tests resulting in wasted time and money. Inability to track patients over time also hindered efforts to develop a standardized longitudinal data base for purposes of conducting studies of clinical outcomes of care. This information could be used for both internal improvement as well as external accountability reporting.

Population-Based Planning

Efforts at clinical integration were also hindered by inadequate population-based planning focused on assessing the health needs of the community and the likely demand for services. Without knowing what the likely demand requirements will be, it is very difficult to determine resource requirements for given services or how those services should be coordinated with each other to provide care of the greatest value. Although the need for such planning was increasingly recognized by the study systems, particularly those operating in Stage 3 and Stage 4 markets with heavier managed care penetration and an increased focus on capitated payment, the systems experienced difficulty obtaining relevant data. National- and state-level data are often inadequate for local market use. Using synthetic estimates also poses problems. In many communities, systems need to collect *primary* data on people's health status, their view of health care facilities and services, and related issues. While the cost of conducting such surveys can be significant, it may be possible to obtain multiple sources of funding by working with the local health department, schools, and private foundations. Useful information can also be obtained from focus groups involving patients and other community members and leaders. Such sessions can at least help identify perceived gaps in services, perceived problems of coordination and continuity of care, and consumer *expectations* regarding the services to be received.

Influence of Market Maturity

As was the case for physician-system integration, the barriers to clinical integration tend to vary as a function of the stage of market maturity, as shown in Table 6.3.

Table 6.3. Barriers to Clinical Integration by Stages of Market Maturity.

Barriers	Stage 1 Unstructured "access" market	Stage 2 "Loose cost" market	Stage 3 Consolidated "advanced cost" market	Stage 4 Strict managed care "value" market
No incentive for clinical integration	++	+	0	0
Institutional autonomy of hospitals	++	++	++	+
Too few physician groups	++	++	++	+
Dispersed geography	0	0	++	+
Lack of a specific strategy or implementation plan for clinical integration	0	0	++	++
Misaligned budgeting, performance appraisal and reward systems	0	0	++	++
Fears of job loss and autonomy threats	0	0	++	++
Information system issues	0	0	++	++
Lack of population-based planning	0	0	++	++

Note: ++ = significant barrier; + = barrier; 0 = usually not a barrier or factor.

In Stage 1 unstructured "access" markets, there is essentially no incentive for clinical integration. This is fortunate, because most systems in these markets are struggling with such issues as the autonomy of individual hospitals and the effort to encourage physicians to participate in more group-like structures. These same factors continue to exist in the Stage 2 "loose cost" markets, except that the economic incentive for clinical integration begins to emerge. Systems must now directly and effectively confront the issues of hospital autonomy and physician group practice formation.

As shown in Table 6.3, it is in the Stage 3 "advanced cost" market that a new and formidable set of clinical integration barriers emerge. These include the previously discussed problems: dispersed geography, lack of a plan to accomplish clinical integration, budgeting, performance appraisal and reward systems that do not reinforce clinical integration activities, fear of job loss and diminished autonomy, information system barriers, and population-based planning challenges. All of these continue to be major issues in the Stage 4 strict managed care "value" market, with the exception of dispersed geography, as regional systems quickly realize the need to form subregions around which more realistic clinical integration expectations can be achieved. As shown, even systems in Stage 4 markets may still struggle with issues of hospital autonomy and physician group practice formation, the latter usually involving consolidation of groups rather than formation.

Key Success Factors and Some Best Practices

The key to successfully creating a clinically integrated continuum of care is the ability to achieve *mass customization* (Davis, 1987; Kotha, 1995). This involves developing services to meet the unique needs of each patient but doing so in an efficient fashion, using relatively standardized support functions that can be applied to all patients and that can coordinate care for all patients across the continuum. Examples of these underlying support processes or capabilities include clinical information systems, multiskilled training, and TQM practices. These represent "across-the-board" investments in the delivery system, creating a common platform from which care can then be tailored as needed to meet the varying needs of patients. These processes represent *robust* investments in that they are likely to be useful to all patients in nearly all circumstances.

The ability to achieve mass customization is very closely tied to the concept of the holographic organization discussed in Chapter Two. The essence of the holographic organization is the ability to embed the "whole" into each "part." In the case of health care, the goal is to have the patient experience each part of the health system as "holistically" as possible in terms of knowledge, expertise, information transfer, and understanding. The individual caregiver is not so much a cog in a wheel but rather is the wheel itself. The "whole" represents the *mass*, which is embedded within the caregiver who then has the capacity to *customize* the service to meet the needs of different patients. In other words, becoming a holographic organization is very much about developing the capacity to mass customize.

Clinical integration helps create the holographic properties needed to realize the community health care management system discussed in Chapter Two. Some of the key factors to successfully address the barriers to clinical integration are highlighted below.

Strategic Factors

As with any organization, the key to health care organizations' efforts to differentiate themselves and succeed in the long run is to develop strategies and capabilities that are difficult for others to imitate (Barney, 1986). This is also important for purposes of collaboration, because in order to be an effective partner, one must bring some distinctive skills or attributes to the table. Developing an aggressive, specific plan for clinical integration is exactly one such strategy. It is difficult for others to imitate because it involves so many variables and barriers, as previously noted. But the present study's evidence suggests that organizations and systems pursuing a *prospector* strategy—characterized by innovation, experimentation, trying to be first or second to the market, and looking for new opportunities—are significantly further along in their clinical integration efforts. Meeting the demands for more cost-effective care means that organizations have to experiment with new ways of delivering care, with efforts to reduce cycle time, and with putting together new kinds of health care teams; they have to retrain workers and care for patients in less costly settings. Attempting to become more efficient *within* current structures and systems—characteristic of a defender strategy—apparently does not work.

To succeed in the health care marketplace requires a specific plan for clinical integration. Such a plan establishes priorities, allocates resources, is accompanied by a specific business plan, and fixes accountability for accomplishment with a specific person. The study systems were beginning to provide such a focus and were charging the system vice president for clinical integration or clinical affairs with responsibility for accomplishment. Mercy Health Services was among the first to develop such a plan, including developing a glossary of key terms associated with the clinical integration concept such as *clinical practice guidelines, community health care system, continuity of care,* and *severity/risk adjustment.*

To have the greatest impact, the clinical integration plan must be linked to population-based planning. Such planning can be contrasted with traditional service-based planning, as shown in Figure 6.1.

Service-based planning takes an "inside-out" approach whereby the organization decides what services it will offer and then organizes and markets care to various patient groups within the population. Typically, these are high-tech services often involving a particular specialty. Examples include infertility clinics, dialysis units, and radiation imaging units.

Population-based planning uses an "outside-in" approach, determining the need for services based on groups of people who may be

Figure 6.1. Traditional Versus Population-Based Planning.

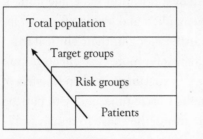

Traditional "inside-out" planning

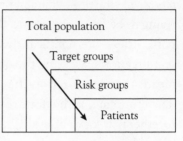

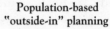

**Population-based
"outside-in" planning**

Source: Jones and Mayerhofer, 1994, pp. 5–6. Figure reprinted with the permission of the publisher.

at risk but who are not currently ill as well as on people living
within a defined geographic service area. Services determined in
this fashion will often cut across the continuum of care and must
be managed within the context of a fixed sum of money.

The outside-in approach thus involves looking not only at past
services and enrolled lives but also at the likely future needs of groups
that may not currently be users of the system's services. Without
some information on community needs, it is difficult to know what
parts of the continuum of care will be most needed, how they might
best be coordinated, or what the service expectations are likely to
be. Lack of such a linkage can result in services being well integrated
from the provider's perspective but not experienced as such by
patients, or in services that don't really address community need.

Fairview was among the study systems more advanced in this
recognition, reflected in the creation of a Department of Community Health. The department routinely conducted community
health needs assessments using focus groups and working groups
with representatives from schools, health departments, youth and
family service agencies, social service and citizen organizations, business organizations, and others. The department was thus able to pri-

oritize needs and develop specific programs to meet those needs. Its work was guided by certain underlying principles, including the following: (1) a broad definition of health, (2) community ownership, (3) shared vision and values, (4) an emphasis on system change, (5) an emphasis on linking initiatives, (6) a neighborhood/regional focus, (7) building competency based on local assets and resources, (8) benchmarking and measuring outcomes, (9) a recognition that things take time, and (10) remembering that there is no single right way (National Civic League, 1995). A second example of population-based planning and implementation from a nonstudy site (Bader, 1995) uses an eight-step approach to identify the major clinical conditions or population groups among its enrollees to target for improvement. The process establishes means to define and/or identify improvement priorities, target populations, desired outcomes, and outcome measures. The belief is that this approach both provides better treatment and controls costs.

Structural Factors

There are several structural factors that can promote clinical integration, including alignment of internal incentives, development of group practices, creation of a clinical effectiveness and outcomes support units, restructuring of patient care, and geographic concentration.

Aligning Internal Incentives

The ability to achieve more clinically integrated care across the continuum must go beyond reorganizing health care professionals into multidisciplinary cross-functional teams working within and across service lines. Such organizational changes must also be accompanied by budgeting, performance appraisal, and reward systems that are based on accomplishing service line objectives. Budgets must be based on service line business plans (for example, cardiovascular, oncology, women's health), with allocation of nursing, supplies, information support, pharmaceutical support, and so on provided to the service line to be managed based on its projected demand for its services. In such cases, the service lines would have some of their own resources for professional development and would not be required to get approval from department-based supervisors.

Performance appraisal needs to be redesigned so that clinical and support personnel are evaluated on accomplishment of team or service line objectives rather than on individual performance standards (Williams, 1992). Greater weight needs to be placed on such skills as the ability to work with and support others, the ability to listen, the willingness to sacrifice for the sake of the team, the ability to use data to arrive at solutions to problems, the ability to manage conflict and change, and the willingness to lead.

Compensation and other rewards based on the performance appraisal system also need to change. Monetary pay and other rewards should be based more on accomplishment of service line objectives than of individual objectives or department- or function-based objectives. For example, some systems were using compensation practices in which base pay was set at the market rate, but bonuses could be earned based on equal achievement of individual goals and team objectives such as shortening length-of-stay or increasing patient satisfaction. Some key points to consider in designing such performance appraisal and compensation systems include (1) involving the input of the team and service line members affected, because they best know the challenges of their jobs; (2) carefully determining what functions and activities are interdependent so as to appropriately fix the scope of responsibility; and (3) ensuring that the targets for achievement are reasonably under the control of team members and yet are set sufficiently high to motivate outstanding performance.

Developing Group Practice

One of the most critical ingredients of clinical integration is developing physician group practices. The Fairview case study presented in Chapter Five illustrates how a system lacking a large multispecialty group such as that of Henry Ford can still create a group-like structure.

Although Fairview physicians practice in 122 different clinics, 50 to 85 percent of primary care patients are under managed care contracts with one network-wide negotiated contract. Fairview provides a number of management and practice support services to FPA. In return, FPA agrees to use Fairview's information systems and to collect productivity, patient satisfaction, clinical outcome, and functional health status data. FPA has enabled Fairview to achieve many of the advantages of a large group practice organization while providing physicians with a sense of autonomy and control over their practices.

Creating a Clinical Effectiveness and Outcomes Support Unit

Improving the coordination of clinical care across the continuum requires analysis of existing processes, development and use of data on current processes and outcomes of care, development of new approaches to care, retraining of personnel, and subsequent evaluation of the redesigned care processes. In addressing these issues, many systems, such as Henry Ford, Advocate, UniHealth, and Mercy, found it necessary to create support units staffed by people with expertise in biostatistics, clinical epidemiology, and related disciplines who could design, conduct, and help interpret the results of various studies. These units were typically composed of three or four people headed by a clinician, who in turn reported directly to a systemwide vice president for clinical integration (the title varies). These units worked with quality improvement project teams and clinical integration task forces, providing data and helping to select problems where existing data could be examined, along with developing primary care data collection instruments. Such units were also closely aligned with the system CQI/TQM activities, either directly incorporating these activities or functioning as part of a larger group reporting to a common person. The support units were engaged in all aspects of clinical data collection and analysis, decision support, guideline, protocol, and pathway development, continuous improvement processes, outcomes measurement, analysis reporting and interpretation, and system redesign work.

Creating such units is an important success factor because personnel directly involved in the caregiving function typically lack the time and all of the needed expertise to do what is required. Caregivers can identify the problem and, of course, be held responsible for implementation, but they must be given resources and support in order to transform clinical processes and better coordinate such processes across the continuum. Systems must make an up-front investment in these units in order to reap advantages in the longer run. Such units also assist in breaking down hospital autonomy barriers to integration by offering all units within the system a "neutral" forum for receiving advice and assistance rather than "forcing" smaller or less influential units to turn to the largest or most influential hospital within the system for advice and assistance.

Restructuring Patient Care

It is impossible to achieve clinical integration without restructuring current patient care practices and, more broadly, the overall approach to preventing disease and promoting health. Figure 6.2 provides a framework for such restructuring.

As shown, the goal—to create healthy communities—begins with an assessment of community needs and preferences. This outside-in approach provides the basis for organizing services, which we suggest involves making three types of decisions: (1) selecting and organizing certain core platform processes; (2) selecting and organizing certain clinical support processes; and (3) selecting and organizing certain direct service lines. *Platform processes and capabilities* refer to those aspects of producing any product or service that cuts across all products or service lines which, if done well, will "raise all boats in the harbor" (Stalk, Evans, and Shulman, 1992). Examples include information systems, registration and scheduling systems, human resources, and planning and marketing functions.

Figure 6.2. Framework for Thinking About Processes.

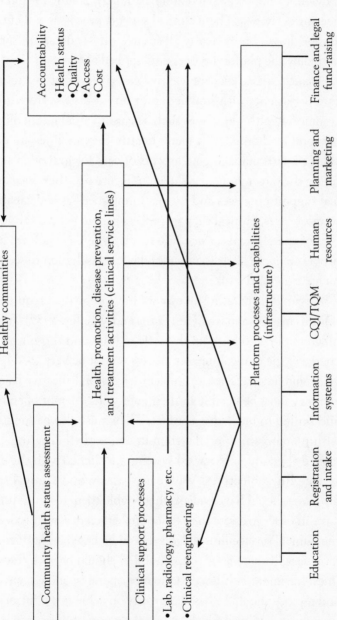

Clinical support processes refer to those functions and activities that directly support the people who directly provide patient care. Obvious examples are laboratory, radiology, pharmacy, and reengineering activities. These clinical support processes will cut across and be drawn on by nearly all service lines, and are in turn supported by the platform processes described above.

Clinical service lines are teams of caregivers organized to provide care to patients with similar conditions or disease states, or with common health objectives such as cardiovascular, oncology, behavioral medicine, or women's health. Service lines are directly charged with managing all aspects of care for individuals constituting the target group. As shown in Figure 6.2, they draw on clinical support processes and the platform processes and capabilities. In most cases, clinical support process people will be active members of the clinical service line teams, whereas platform process people are more likely to provide ad hoc consultation to such teams on an as-needed basis.

Organizing care in the way we have described requires great skills in matrix management (Burns and Wholey, 1989). In particular, people who head up the service lines and those who are in charge of the clinical support processes must be very good listeners and communicators, astute problem solvers, and effective team players; they must be flexible in their approach, tolerant of ambiguity, and skilled in managing conflict. They must also be functioning within an organizational system in which the budgeting, performance appraisal, and reward systems are aligned with the clinical service line objectives. Whereas platform and clinical support processes should have budgets that enable them to determine their costs in order to assess their functional efficiency and productivity, the clinical service line budgets should be based on both costs *and revenue.* Ultimate fiscal accountability should be with the service lines. In similar fashion, performance appraisal and compensation and rewards should be based primarily on achieving clinical service line objectives even for the clinical support and platform process personnel. In several study systems, incentive or bonus pay was increasingly based on achieving service line and larger organizational objectives above and beyond meeting support or platform process goals.

Organizing care around core processes also requires identifying rules or guidelines for *combining* services, functions, and activities. The underlying criteria to consider are the degree of interdependence or relatedness of the services, functions, or activities under consideration. Three potentially useful guidelines suggest that services, functions, and activities can be combined if they are (1) clinically related, (2) socio-demographically linked, or (3) organizationally related.

Following the guideline of clinical relatedness means combining activities that involve similar treatment inputs, practices, and approaches. This is, of course, one of the primary criteria used for determining clinical service lines and would be particularly prevalent in the area of high-technology acute care services.

Another guideline to consider is the socio-demographic composition of the population to be served. Using such demographic characteristics as age, sex, ethnicity, or income, service lines may be organized around women, senior citizens, Hispanic Americans, African Americans, or people with low incomes. Organizing around socio-demographic characteristics of the community will be more prevalent when dealing with primary care, disease prevention, and health promotion issues.

The third guideline is to consider the organizational demands or requirements of the activity. These include the organizational structure, the skill mix of personnel, and various logistical issues. The goal here is to achieve managerial economies of scope such that the current structure, personnel, and logistical support services are used to their best advantage.

Sometimes one guideline will predominate, as in the case of cardiovascular disease, where the clinical approach for combining services will come to the forefront. In other cases, combinations of guidelines may be used, as in the case of breast cancer screening programs for women of targeted age groups. In other circumstances, the guidelines may be in conflict with each other, as in the case of those who believe educational programs involving AIDS patients should be part of an overall community health educational initiative versus those who believe the programs ought to be targeted for separate attention. The goal in all cases, however, should be to organize care such that patients and community members experience the most continuous care possible with the best achievable outcomes using the fewest resources. Inevitably, there will be some trade-offs across patient groups and community members because achieving cost-effective care for the greatest number of people is the goal and challenge of mass customization.

Fairview Southdale Hospital provides one example in its effort to combine services, functions, and activities by distinguishing between inpatient services and two types of ambulatory services. Type I ambulatory procedures are those that are relatively routine and predictable. They are not likely to result in complications and are not tied to an inpatient facility (Allen and Weber, 1995). Some examples include knee arthroscopy, many ENT procedures, D and Cs, and mammography. Organizational criteria of efficiency in scheduling procedures, billing, and capacity utilization are likely to be most important with this group.

In contrast, Type II ambulatory procedures are more complex and less predictable. They vary in time and are subject to more complications. Examples include cholecystectomies, hernia repairs, hysterectomies, CT scans, angiography, cardiac-catheterizations, and MRIs. The unpredictability of many of these procedures requires the availability of inpatient care as a backup in case of complications and as a short-term option for patients that might need extended observation. Thus, for these procedures and conditions, clinical criteria for grouping take priority over organizational criteria, and these services need to be located closer to inpatient units. But at the same time, Fairview recognizes that there is an interdependency between

Type I and II ambulatory services in that many physicians perform both types of procedures. Thus, by sharing personnel, technology, and administrative assistance between both types, economies of scope and potentially of scale can be realized. This argues for a "health care campus" concept in which Type I and Type II ambulatory and inpatient care services are located closely together.

There are many examples of successful patient care restructuring. At the level of acute and intensive care, more services are being brought to the patient's bedside, such as respiratory therapy, radiology, and laboratory services. These are designed to shorten cycle times, reduce the probability of communication errors, and eliminate patient transfers (Lathrop, 1993; Weber and Weber, 1994). Nurses and other caregivers are being trained in a greater number and variety of skills. In one case, this resulted in a more than 50 percent cut in the number of staff members seen by a patient (Lathrop, 1993, p. 193). At Sentara Health System, all employees are classified as administrative, clinical, or service, and are cross-trained— within licensure constraints—to perform various treatments such as phlebotomy and respiratory therapy (Weber and Weber, 1994). Diagnostic facilities are equipped with multipurpose rooms where a variety of tests are conducted without having the patients go from room to room.

At the New England Medical Center in Boston, adult and pediatric hematology/oncology services and cardiac care services were redesigned to improve continuity of care. This redesign included rotating nurses between inpatient and outpatient care; installing computers in patients' homes for ready communication with physicians, nurses, and other families having similar problems; developing a clinical information system with a common data base for all persons to track treatment plans; and creating a new care coordinator position (Weber and Weber, 1994). The changes have resulted in significant improvements in nursing care continuity, increases in the number of patients who stay in only one unit within the hospital, shorter lengths of stay, and more accurate communication between doctors and nurses (O'Brien, Shortell, and Hughes, 1994). Similar results have also been found in Veterans Administration hospitals (Smith, 1995).

It is important to note that the *degree* of patient care restructuring required to support clinical integration efforts is largely a function of the market stage the organization is in (see Table 6.3), the nature of current structures and approaches to care, and people's ability to change. Often, restructuring work will progress through three stages: (1) process restructuring and redesign; (2) information technology–based redesign; and (3) comprehensive operational and organizational redesign (Smith-Daniels, Schweikhart, and Kronenfeld, 1994). Process restructuring and redesign largely builds on the organization's CQI/TQM efforts. It emphasizes the redefinition of work roles, development of multidisciplinary teams, streamlining of top management, and development of a group-oriented culture emphasizing participation. The information technology–intensive approach highlights reengineering efforts (that is, eliminating entire processes) and is typically a more radical departure from what was going on before. It involves a greater commitment of time and resources. The comprehensive approach brings together all elements of restructuring—culture, work roles, information and production technologies, and redesign of physical facilities—to create greater continuity of care and value for patients. By the time an organization or health system finds itself in a mature Stage 4 market, it had better be achieving comprehensive care redesign, or it will be operating from a competitive disadvantage.

Patient care restructuring is necessary for clinical integration, but it alone is insufficient. In fact, an argument can be made that such restructuring can serve as a *barrier* to clinical integration and is therefore not only unnecessary but also possibly dangerous! The problem is that almost all patient care restructuring efforts undertaken to date have centered on acute inpatient care and a limited number of diseases or conditions. While a few efforts have extended across the continuum of care to include home care and post acute care, these efforts have still focused on acute care as the center of the redesign effort as opposed to the community, the patient, or the primary care physician. In fact, an argument could be made that the net result of all the patient-focused care restructuring hyperactivity of the past five years has been to *increase the fragmentation* of health care in the United States. The same can be said for advocates of disease stage management (Lumsdon, 1995). They have created highly integrated specialized care units organized around a few diseases, units that are linked neither to each other nor to the broader issues of providing community-focused care across the continuum. We have solved one problem only to create and exacerbate others. The issue, however, is not patient-focused care or disease stage management but rather the breadth of their application and, perhaps, the breadth of vision of their advocates to date. The lessons and principles of patient-focused care and disease stage management need to be placed within the larger framework of population-based health care planning and within the outside-in paradigm of system thinking, which begins with the community, moves on to various target groups and, ultimately, to specific services.

But more is needed than a broadened vision and a wider planning paradigm. The *system* of care itself, however restricted, must be managed and governed differently. A fundamental lesson all the study systems learned is that you cannot ask physicians, nurses, and other health professionals to produce more team-based, data-based, outcome-based care while still operating with an old, outmoded management and governance structure. The system of care must be managed and governed differently. This is so important a success factor that it is accorded special treatment in Chapter Seven.

Geographic Concentration

Services and facilities must be located close enough together to be physically able to create a clinically integrated continuum of care. As previously noted, we found that systems that were so spread out that care sites were an average of fifty miles or more apart from each other scored significantly lower on almost all clinical integration measures, including shared clinical service lines, protocols, and outcome measures. There are limits to both patients' and physicians' willingness to travel. Primary care practices, multispecialty practices, diagnostic clinics, acute care units, home health services, nursing homes, hospices, and other services must be located or made available in reasonable contiguity to each other to facilitate transport across sites as needed. It is also easier to bring people from different units of a system together in order to learn from each other and share best practices when they are geographically closer to each other. Recognizing this, several systems, such as Advocate, Henry Ford, Sutter, UniHealth, Sisters of Providence, and Franciscan, even though based in highly populated urban areas, created several subregional systems to serve as focal points for integration activities, particularly for those relating to clinical integration. The challenge to the corporate system support office is to take the best practices and lessons learned within each of the subregions and ensure that they are diffused across the entire system to benefit all.

Cultural Factors

The cultural factors most critical to clinical integration are commitment to CQI/TQM, training of multiskilled workers, and development of physician leadership.

CQI/TQM Commitment

Although CQI/TQM itself contains strategic, structural, cultural, and technical components (Shortell, Levin, and others, 1995; O'Brien, Shortell, and others, 1995), we believe CQI/TQM's dominant role in clinical integration work is to provide an overall cultural mindset to the enterprise. The key is its emphasis on empowering those individuals closest to the direct provision of patient care to take responsibility for continuously improving their work and providing them with the authority and tools to do so. The emphasis is on understanding and streamlining underlying processes to improve quality and outcomes of care rather than on blaming individuals. The emphasis is on defining, understanding, and meeting customer needs instead of accommodating professional needs. These emphases represent a cultural shift for health care organizations, which typically emphasize personal physician responsibility and control over patient care; there is a reluctance to delegate or to experiment and a tendency to punish individual outliers.

CQI/TQM also provides a common language for improvement. Every system studied indicated that exposing people to the training, philosophies, and practices of CQI/TQM was critical for engaging in clinical integration work. It helped to provide the medium through which people could communicate with each other, gather and analyze data on what services might best be combined, decide on the most efficient series of steps for providing the service, and develop process and outcome measures for assessing performance. CQI/TQM was used by Fairview and Sentara, for example, to develop protocols for coronary bypass graft surgery that resulted in a four-day length of stay for Fairview and a three-day protocol for Sentara. Nearly every system made frequent use of cross-functional multidisciplinary teams to coordinate care across the continuum for patients experiencing problems of congestive heart failure, substance abuse, orthopedic surgery, oncology, and obstetrics. In the past four years alone, Henry Ford has trained over 3,500 physicians and employees in TQM practices and principles with 500 of these (including 250 physicians) having received a six-day introductory course. This has served as the foundation for their clinical integration and clinical process improvement work in a variety of areas, including cervical cancer screening, laboratory testing, joint replacement, obstetrics, and asthma care. As noted by one Ford employee, "Today it's hard to imagine significant progress in improving clinical services without this cultural shift supported by total quality management." (Henry Ford Health System, 1993).

Fairview's clinical integration work has been based in large part on five CQI core beliefs: (1) focus on individual leadership, (2) focus on customers, (3) focus on process, (4) focus on people, and

(5) focus on measurement. These beliefs have been translated into behavioral examples for every employee, and each employee's performance is measured by how effectively he or she has demonstrated the belief in action on a seven-point scale, where one equals ineffective and seven equals effective. Examples of ineffective performance include "fails to understand how actions and decisions affect others' work or business as a whole," "focuses only on traditional areas of responsibility," "operates independent from the team," and "resists the input and assistance from others." Examples of positive behavior include "takes a systematic approach to resolving problems and issues," "recognizes that customer needs and expectations extend beyond department boundaries," "seeks to remove processes not required to meet customer expectations," and "functions as an integral team member." The cases studies later in this chapter provide further examples of CQI/TQM as a key success factor in achieving meaningful levels of clinical integration.

New Training for New Workers

Clinical integration depends on developing multiskilled workers who take a holistic view of the patient and of the continuum of care required to maintain, enhance, or restore the patient's health. Although this could just as easily be considered a technical success factor, the key again is the cultural value of wholeness, integration, and empowerment. Multiskilled professionals who can operate in teams, with a clear focus on customer requirements, contribute to developing the holographic organization (see Chapter Two) in which the whole is embedded in each part. Several systems were making major efforts in cross-training as part of their CQI/TQM and clinical reengineering work. For example, Sharp instituted a centralized employment unit in which new hirees receive training in CQI/TQM, exposure to Sharp's mission and values, and, to the extent possible, are provided multiple skills to function in a variety of direct patient care, clinical support, and administrative support activities throughout the system. These individuals regard themselves as Sharp HealthCare employees, *not* employees of an individual unit or group.

An important feature of multiskilled training is adopting a philosophy of *continuous learning*. The organizations furthest along in the cross-training and multiskilled training used every opportunity that arose in the course of doing daily work as an opportunity for learning. Reports on "lessons learned" were built into every team meeting. Great reliance was placed on developing self-teaching modules. Performance appraisal criteria were developed in which an individual did not receive credit for learning a new skill until he or she had taught it or shared it with someone else. Incentives for participating in advanced CQI/TQM training were created whereby individuals only received credit if *all* team or unit members attended. These represent examples of building the "learning organization" (Senge, 1990; Huber and Glick, 1993) essential to clinical integration. Such activities were not limited to nurses and other health professionals but were also directed at physicians, often taking the form of retraining subspecialty internists into comprehensive primary care physicians. An example of how such training and learning works at the micro level is highlighted below.

> [Developing guidelines] is a complex process. It involves training and forms revision and reconfiguration of scheduling and information systems—an enormous number of activities. In our system, this process involves some 5,000 front line and support staff. Hundreds of daily encounters occur in 50 locations, each with its own ways of scheduling, of handling what patient information is dispensed, how it's dispensed, how nurses and doctors interact, who does what.
>
> For example, suppose you want to implement the bladder infection protocol. You go to the physician's office and you sit down with the nurse and the doctor who [is] in a larger practice with five doctors and a couple of

nurses and the receptionist—and you ask, "What's your current process for managing a bladder infection?"

There is a little pause, and the head nurse looks at you and says, "For which doctor?"

And then you say "Well, let's pick Dr. Jones." And she says, "Well, Dr. Jones is fairly new here, and he set up a system with these little three by five cards. We've got them in a box by the phone. We just look up bladder infection, and here's what it says: 'Come in, given a urinalysis and culture. See the doctor.'"

So how do you usually put this guideline to work in a pre-existing system like this one? You use what you've got. You embed the guideline on that three by five card. If they've got some other kind of system—computer scheduling system reminders—you incorporate it there. That's the key to making it happen. That's what "do" is all about.

That same process has to happen for literally every physician throughout the system of 50 different practices. A lot of people's time is taken up in these difficult labor intensive implementation activities. That's where we have to count on the commitment and motivation of the medical groups and the organizations. . . .

Why do physicians and nurses take this on, and what keeps them going? It's not money, because we don't add a lot of money to the system for this. I think what keeps people doing this is that we start to generate an interesting learning engine. Physicians and nurses are trained scientifically, and many of them harbor a lot of curiosity. Does what they do in practice work or doesn't it?

This process is giving them a mechanism to start answering some questions that they wondered about for 20 years of practice. I wouldn't minimize the importance of this kind of motivation. It's what's going to sustain us over the long haul. [Reinertsen, 1994, pp. 58–59.]

Physician Leadership Development

The importance of physician leadership development and suggestions for promoting it were discussed in Chapter Five. It is sufficient to note here the special role physician leadership plays in promoting clinical integration. The goal is to develop physician leaders who understand patient care from a population-based perspective, who understand patients from a holistic perspective, who understand care delivery from a continuum of care perspective, who understand and are able to operate in teams and promote teamwork throughout the organization, and who understand how to use information systems to promote clinical integration work and to develop outcome measures for both continuous improvement and external accountability purposes. Almost all systems were incorporating content in each of the above areas into their leadership development programs. In the case of Henry Ford, this was being done in a highly experiential way, using current clinical integration issues facing physicians in their practices as the focus for application.

Technical Factors

Three major technical factors help to promote clinical integration: information systems, reengineering, and joint education.

Information Systems

We discuss the importance of information systems as a key to successful physician-system integration (Chapter Five) and as being at the center of community health system management activities associated with the "capability wheel" (Chapter Two). Information systems are needed that would link national data on effectiveness, outcomes, and "best practices" for given conditions with each system's own efforts to develop protocols and pathways of care, to continuously improve processes, to reengineer work, and to monitor and evaluate improvement interventions. Some keys to developing such information systems appear to be to (1) focus on the information needs of providers and patients associated with primary care and home care, since this is where the largest volume of transactions occur, rather than organizing the system around acute inpatient hospital care; (2) develop a core module that is likely to be used by all caregivers and that will be drawn on not only by internal caregivers but also external agencies (for example, patient demographics, diagnoses, complications); (3) build in flexible modules that can be tailored to the special needs of different caregivers (for example, pharmacists, nurses, home health agency personnel, hospice personnel, and physicians); (4) develop and identify data that "follow" the patient throughout the continuum of care; and (5) develop the capability to take individual encounter data and aggregate them across individuals by diagnoses, comorbidities, patient characteristics, treatment settings, caregivers, and so on, in order to conduct effectiveness and outcome studies on a retrospective, concurrent, and prospective basis.

Reengineering

Reengineering involves a fundamental "starting over" (Hammer and Champy, 1993), a willingness to consider eliminating entire processes, programs, and services. As such, it has an important cultural component, but we choose to discuss it as a technical success factor because of the demands it places on the organization's technical core: its production processes, competencies, and capabilities. Reengineering and CQI/TQM are related in that they try to better meet customer needs and improve organizational performance, but they are also somewhat different. Reengineering, in a sense, goes beyond CQI/TQM by recognizing that some processes, programs, and services may require more than continuous improvement of existing behavior or reductions in variation; namely, they may require total elimination and redesign. The difference is largely a matter of degree, but that difference is important because reengineering often runs into more vocal and heated political opposition within the organization. The scope of change is often much more pervasive in reengineering than in most CQI/TQM initiatives.

A number of study systems found that in order to promote more clinically integrated care, entire processes, functions, departments, and categories of personnel would need to be eliminated. For example, Sentara eliminated the hospital's Department of Physical Therapy; these functions were reassigned to nurses and other therapists. Some physical therapists were reassigned to primary care in home health teams. A pharmaceutical redesign project resulted in the elimination of the inpatient pharmacy department and the redeployment of pharmaceutical service managers, who used their skills to help manage patients across the care continuum. Other examples exist in the literature, including Lee Memorial Hospital in Fort Myers, Florida; it reengineered its orthopedic and related services, which resulted in a 35 percent drop in patient accidents and $2.2 million in savings (Kennedy, 1994).

There appear to be three keys to successful reengineering efforts. The first is for the organization to have some experience with CQI/TQM. No health care organization has successfully achieved reengineering without it. Second, it is important to select core processes for reengineering work if one expects to achieve demonstrable improvement in clinical integration and any possible attendant cost reductions. In other fields, for example, it is estimated that reengineering a minor process or single activity has only a 1 percent effect on the bottom line; reengineering a core process or several interdependent processes can realize a 3 to 5 percent payoff; reengineering the entire organization might have as much as a 17 percent effect (Hall, Rosenthal, and Wade, 1993). Third, there is the need for strong information system technologies that contain key features: open architecture, the ability to network, and data base design (Kralovec, 1994). Reengineering exploits a health care organization's information strengths. Those organizations that report some success in their reengineering efforts appear to be those with a more advanced ability to manage information, such as the Henry Ford and Intermountain Health systems (Griffith, Sahney, and Mohr, 1995).

Joint Education

Clinical integration requires practice both on and off the field. It is a team sport. As long as physicians, nurses, executives, and other health professionals continue to conduct their own seminars, conferences, and symposia with little mutual involvement, clinical integration progress will be slow and uneven. The key is to educate the team. Some of this needs to take place "off the field," laying the groundwork for what clinical integration is and what core competencies are required for achieving it. But a lot needs to take place "on the field" in the heat of battle, through learning by doing. The key is constant vigilance, awareness, and monitoring of results of the team efforts. The problem is not in making mistakes but in failing to learn from them. Greater emphasis must be placed on real-time learning if health care organizations are to make significant advances in their clinical integration efforts. The study systems with a more group-oriented, developmental culture (see Chapter Three), with greater experience of CQI/TQM and with more fully developed information systems, generally appear to be further along in their ability to transfer learning throughout the system in pursuit of their clinical integration objectives.

Characteristics of a Mature Clinically Integrated System

Ultimately, clinical integration should result in more cost-effective patient care as might be measured by cost per episode of illness for prevalent conditions in the community and such ratios as cost per disability day prevented and quality-adjusted life year. Until such measures and analysis tools are available, however, reliance must be placed on intermediate measures: reductions in missed appointments, elimination of duplicate testing, shorter turnaround times for tests, less unnecessary repeating of questions for patients, increased patient satisfaction, increased continuity of care, and related indicators. In order to chart progress on becoming more clinically integrated, one can also draw on the structure and process indicators used in the present study pertaining to shared clinical protocols and pathways, shared use of outcome measures, common patient identifiers, shared clinical service lines, and shared clinical support services (Devers and others, 1994).

In addition to quantifiable outcome measures and tracking methodologies, we believe there are certain intangible characteristics of more mature clinically integrated systems. These are highlighted in the list that follows.

Characteristics of a Mature Clinically Integrated System

- Knows the health needs of its communities.

- Knows the resources required across the continuum of care to address these needs.

- Knows what it can provide itself, and what it can provide in partnership with others.

- Knows its work. Knows the caregiving processes required across the continuum of care to promote, enhance, maintain, and restore health in a cost-effective fashion.

- "Knows that it knows." Knows what it knows and what it does not know. Is a self-aware organization with a growing capacity to learn.

- Knows how to get better and how to adapt to changing circumstances. Has processes and methods for improvement.

- Continually invests in its human capital.

- Is able to consistently meet stakeholder expectations.

Most of these have been discussed in previous chapters. Perhaps the most important characteristic, however—the one that would clearly distinguish the more advanced systems from the less advanced—is the ability to *consistently* meet stakeholder expectations. It is relatively easy for any organization or system to fully meet customer needs on any given occasion. But what distinguishes excellent organizations is their ability to do so time after time, with every customer they encounter and with their suppliers, partners, and external groups. Such consistency is extremely difficult to achieve in any industry or circumstance but is particularly difficult for service organizations that must deal with the reactions of people being served. Individuals' tastes and preferences change, and in the case of health care one must also deal with each person's unique response—physiological and emotional—to illness. Staff turnover, organizational restructuring, clinical reengineering, mergers and acquisitions, and strategic alliance activity can all be terribly disruptive of efforts to achieve more clinically integrated care for patients. Ironically, many of these same activities are intended to achieve greater clinical integration! The mature clinically integrated organizations will be those that sink their roots a little deeper; that learn their lessons a little quicker; that transfer the lessons to others more rapidly; and that embed a wider vision and mental model of health care delivery into each of its people. Each person becomes a mini comprehensive health care system.

Such a system will also know what clinical integration structures work best for itself. It will know how to identify high-leverage clinical integration initiatives, how to launch systemwide initiatives, and how to identify the key ingredients that cut across all clinical integration work. The structures will help identify resource and data requirements based on in-depth knowledge of the core processes underlying a coordinated continuum of care. High-leverage initiatives will be based on those likely to yield the greatest value to, and have the most pervasive impact on, the health of the populations served. Systemwide initiatives will be closely linked to strategic priorities that achieve specific clinical integration objectives. Visible, accountable leadership; built-in communication, education, and training; ongoing improvement strategies; and performance appraisal and reward systems—all are aligned with the overall effort. Finally, the key ingredients that cut across all clinical integration work are those strategic, structural, cultural, and technical success factors we have highlighted in this chapter. The three case studies that follow provide illustrations.

Henry Ford Health System

When the study began, Henry Ford Health System (HFHS) could be characterized as having limited clinical integration. Although pockets of excellence existed throughout the system, these successful efforts were not coordinated or communicated effectively across the system. No formal plan for achieving clinical integration was evident nor was there a commonly accepted definition of clinical integration. Tensions among the various groups of physicians practicing at HFHS inhibited clinical integration. Clinical integration efforts tended to be inpatient focused with relatively little outpatient component. Overall, HFHS's clinical integration efforts had no coherence and thus were not as effective as they might otherwise be.

Progress Toward Clinical Integration at HFHS

During the study period, Henry Ford Health System made important strides toward clinical integration in a number of areas, including some reorganization of the delivery system, improvement of clinical processes, performance measurement initiatives, reengineering of primary care, and early steps toward meaningful population-based planning. Many of these specific initiatives are tied together by a growing system-level focus on health status through health maintenance, disease prevention, and improved management of chronic illness. Some of the initiatives and activities are targeted at the delivery-system level and others at the hospital or medical group level.

Henry Ford Health System has a number of key initiatives and activities focused on the delivery-system level. For example, in order to increase the system's responsiveness to its customers at the local level, Henry Ford is realigning its organization structure regionally. Coordination of patient care and management of spending will be regional responsibilities, while some product lines (for example, hemodialysis, home health care) will be organized on a systemwide basis. The Delivery System Design Team is charged with developing the system's organizational model for delivering health care services and identifying the tasks associated with implementation. This includes defining the system's regions, the infrastructure, and the business groups operating within the system.

The delivery system is also being affected by the integration of the system's two group practices. Metro Medical Group (MMG) and the Henry Ford Medical Group (HFMG) started as separate entities with different reporting structures and policies, and sometimes tension existed between the two. However, these two groups have recently merged. The MMG staff and facilities have been integrated into the HFMG and the overall system regional organizational structure with the aim of improving customer service and operational efficiency.

HFHS pursues improvement of clinical care processes in the context of an ongoing TQM effort. The System-wide Clinical Practice Improvement Initiative is a three-phase, fifteen-month process that aims to assure uniform and consistent value in health care services delivered to every HFHS customer. This process will redesign the infrastructure and processes required to support systemwide clinical practice improvement. As part of Phase I, locally developed initiatives —focused on childbirth care and adult asthma management—are being implemented systemwide. Partnership in Pregnancy and Parenting is an innovative approach that links perinatal education, an intensive third-trimester maternal assessment, and two postpartum home health visits with a shortened inpatient length of stay. This approach has reduced length of stay while maintaining high patient satisfaction and clinical quality. The Adult Asthma Management Program is based on the clinical guideline for asthma developed by the National Institutes for Health. Under this guideline, patients are provided education on self-management, including instruction in the use of a peak flow meter to measure their own breathing. The program aims to improve the ability of adult asthmatics to self-monitor and self-manage, under the supervision of their primary care providers, so they experience fewer asthma symptoms and treatment side effects. As a result, they require treatment less often, and asthma-related ER visits and admissions decline.

Three other initiatives are also aimed at promoting high-quality, consistent clinical decision making. The System Radiology Reporting Initiative links all main hospital campus sites and outpatient locations where radiology services are provided through the radiology information system, making it possible to track process steps, results, and patient folders. The System Laboratory Initiative seeks to ensure uniform clinical and service standards—comprehensive, high quality, and cost-effective—by integrating the system's laboratories, which have traditionally functioned separately. Similarly, the Unified Formulary Initiative seeks to develop a standard of prescribing practice for all HFHS entities.

The Managed Care College is a year-long program designed to help prepare HFMG clinicians and administrators function in the managed care arena. The curriculum includes such subjects as clinical decision making, outcomes management, and CQI. The college currently has two curricular tracks. The first seeks to provide HFMG leadership with skills to promote primary care development and managed care orientation. The second "clinical practice" track concentrates on improving clinical care, especially in ambulatory settings. Participants in both of these tracks spend at least fifty hours in the classroom.

HFHS is developing a number of mechanisms to aid the communication and coordination of system efforts. For example, the Center for Health Promotion and Disease Prevention was created to support and foster coordination among the many existing system (as well as community) health promotion activities. Leadership HFHS is a new program that seeks to promote awareness of the various functions and roles within the system. Forty-three employees, selected from fifteen units within the system, meet monthly to share their experiences and learn from each other. The full-day sessions include discussion with system leaders and active participation in various system settings.

Clinical integration within HFHS is also furthered by a consistent and growing emphasis on performance measurement. Leaders of HFHS recognize the importance of developing measures of all major dimensions of performance and moving beyond such traditional measures as occupancy rates, length of stay, financial ratios, and production statistics. HFHS is moving toward meaningful performance measurement in four main areas: customer service, low-cost provider, system integration, and growth (see Figure 6.3).

Measuring performance in these four areas holds the promise of permitting development of a comprehensive system performance profile.

HFHS is involved in two important performance measurement initiatives. Led by the Center for Clinical Effectiveness and in conjunction with a national effort by the American Group Practice Association, the Henry Ford Medical Group is collecting and evaluating health status data on patients with diabetes, hip replacement, asthma, and hypertension. There are also plans to add low back pain to the set of clinical conditions under study. The ultimate goal is to expand this type of health status assessment to the entire HFHS patient population.

A second important performance measurement effort is the Consortium Research on Indicators of System Performance (CRISP). Led by HFHS researchers, this ongoing project seeks to develop a more appropriate and comprehensive measurement system for vertically integrated health systems. The goal is to produce a set of performance indicators that give a truly comprehensive picture, or "balanced scorecard," of system performance.

Figure 6.3. System Performance Measurement.

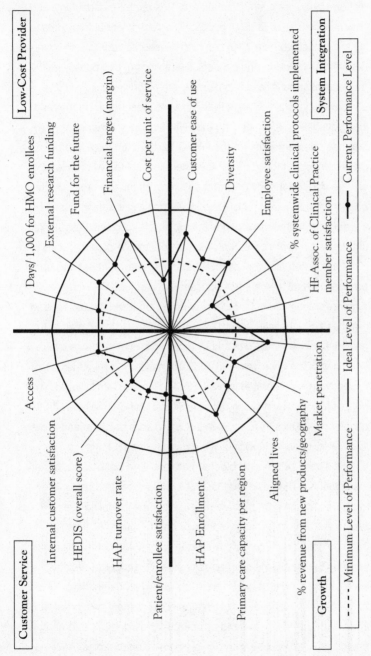

Low-Cost Provider

System Integration

Customer Service

Growth

Financial target (margin)
Cost per unit of service
External research funding
Days/1,000 for HMO enrollees
Fund for the future
Customer ease of use
Diversity
Employee satisfaction
% systemwide clinical protocols implemented
HF Assoc. of Clinical Practice member satisfaction
Market penetration
% revenue from new products/geography
Aligned lives
Primary care capacity per region
HAP Enrollment
Patient/enrollee satisfaction
HAP turnover rate
HEDIS (overall score)
Internal customer satisfaction
Access

- - - - Minimum Level of Performance ——— Ideal Level of Performance ——●—— Current Performance Level

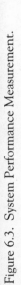

Note: The diagram shown is for illustrative purposes only and does not reflect actual performance.
Source: Henry Ford Health System. Reprinted with permission.

HFHS facilitates clinical integration by taking steps toward population-based planning. Biostatistics, Research Epidemiology, and Medical Informatics (BREMI) began the collection of outcome data to lay the groundwork for such planning. Resources committed to this department included one biomedical statistician, two public health–trained statisticians, and two health systems analysts.

Several initiatives and activities have concentrated on the medical group level. Reengineering the HFMG primary care delivery system has been a priority for the HFMG for the past three years. The Saturn Project of the Internal Medicine Clinic at Henry Ford Hospital was an important early care process innovation. The project's purpose was to redesign patient service in the clinical setting based on a team approach. Teams of physicians, nurses, physician assistants, and technicians are collectively responsible for the care of panels of patients. The team approach enhances patients' access to care because several members of the team may be qualified and available to address the patients' problems at any given time. The project also emphasizes a holistic approach to patients, addressing all of the patients' issues rather than focusing narrowly on medical problems.

Many of the improvements and lessons learned from the Saturn Project were incorporated into the HFMG Primary Care Initiative. The goal of this effort, involving physicians and staff from all the HFMG primary care clinics, is to improve the way care is delivered and make it easier for patients to receive the care they need. Efforts have identified a series of building blocks that rest on a base of customer expectations. The basic foundation blocks are panels (that is, aligning patients with primary care physicians), a scheduling system, a phone system, and primary/specialty collaboration. All these foundation blocks are necessary to reach the top block of the pyramid, which is the HFMG vision of primary care. A number of projects for each of the foundation blocks have resulted in alignment of about 65 percent of all HFMG patients with a personal primary care physician, improved phone service and appointment availability, and an improved referral process from primary care to orthopedics. As these foundation blocks are being built and strengthened, HFMG is also working on higher blocks in the pyramid, including service recovery, nursing advice, guidelines, open access, and managing care. (A similar initiative has recently been launched for specialty care.)

Reengineering also involves dissemination of primary care clinical guidelines and greater use of nonphysician providers whenever appropriate, thereby reducing the cost of care and improving access. HFHS also created primary care councils to enhance primary care performance. The primary care council for pediatrics, for example, brings together heads of areas and clinical sites to determine priorities, resolve problems, and institute changes. Similar councils exist for adult primary care and emergency medicine.

A second initiative focusing on the medical group level is the Ambulatory Practice Improvement Program structure, which aims to integrate clinical practice improvement activities into daily work in all Henry Ford medical centers. HFMG has historically been inconsistent in its reporting and oversight of quality assessment and improvement activities in ambulatory care. The Ambulatory Practice Improvement Program structure is designed to standardize measures as well as to establish mechanisms of assessment and dissemination of information. In addition, lines of responsibility are clearly identified.

Obstacles to Clinical Integration

Clinical integration efforts at Henry Ford Health System have occurred despite the presence of barriers to integration. In fact, many of the efforts detailed above seem to be a direct response to the identified barriers. Some of the barriers discussed below are inherent in the system's approach to clinical integration, whereas others stem from broader characteristics of the system as a whole.

At the most basic level, clinical integration was slowed by the absence of a formal clinical integration plan or a commonly accepted definition of clinical integration within the system. In addition, clinical integration activities at the system and subregional levels have not always been coordinated and communicated effectively across the system. Many worthwhile projects have been undertaken, but often people in the system other than those immediately involved in the project have had little or no knowledge of such efforts. However, problems of conceptual and operational clarity in regard to clinical integration have diminished within the medical group with the Primary Care Initiative and the Ambulatory Practice Improvement Program Structure as well as within the primary care councils in pediatrics, adult medicine, and emergency medicine. In addition, specific clinical integration responsibilities have been assigned to specific people, which helps give coherence to the clinical integration effort. The development of the Delivery System Design Team—with its focus on the configuration, roles, and responsibilities of the regions as well as on what constitutes systemwide clinical product lines—has helped resolve some of the coordination and communication problems within the system as a whole. The Center for Health Promotion and Disease Prevention is working to coordinate the system's health promotion activities and its focus on community health status.

Another barrier to full-scale clinical integration has been an almost exclusive focus on inpatient care processes in the development of clinical pathways and protocols. Most of the protocols developed at HFHS in the name of clinical integration have covered only a limited continuum of care, with little if any outpatient component. Most protocols developed within HFHS have also had limited horizontal integration across units at the same level within the system. Protocols developed at one hospital have not been routinely shared with the relevant actors at other hospitals within the system. However, these problems are being addressed through a number of mechanisms, such as the System-wide Clinical Practice Improvement Initiative. Guidelines now being developed span a much wider spectrum of the continuum of care. In addition, councils and task forces involved in clinical integration activities are much more likely to be cross-continuum, multidisciplinary, and multisite.

Broader system characteristics impeding clinical integration include tensions among the system's various physician groups, physician attitudes, underdeveloped information systems, and inappropriate incentives built into the system's primary financing vehicle. Significant tension has existed between the group practices, now merged, and between them and private physicians with patients in the system. These tensions have tended to reduce physicians' effectiveness in clinical integration efforts. For example, physicians in the smaller group practice and the pool of private physicians have often been reluctant to accept clinical pathways developed by the larger medical group. Physicians in the larger medical group also have had the reputation (with other system physicians) of being "know-it-alls," of lacking a customer orientation, of having teaching and research conflicts, and of having low tolerance for "average" physicians. Private physicians within the system appear to have an inappropriate fear of this medical group. However, the merger of HFHS's two major medical groups (MMG and HFMG) has helped to remedy many of these problems. The eventual outcome is not yet known, but the merger has been proceeding with surprising speed and smoothness. And the system is trying to get private physicians more involved.

Unsupportive physician attitudes have also posed challenges for clinical integration. In the past, the system lacked a sufficient number of physician champions of the clinical integration concept. However, HFHS now has many more physician leaders and champions thanks to its development efforts. HFHS still encounters the unwillingness of private physicians to commit time, making it difficult to integrate them into the clinical integration process. These private physicians usually also have little or no CQI education, making it difficult to include them in integration efforts that are grounded in the CQI approach. The system is attempting to deal with this problem in a number of ways. There is some discussion of including private physicians in the Managed Care College. In addition, some private physicians have been trained "just in time" by hospital quality staff and are participating in or leading some quality improvement efforts.

Clinical integration has also been delayed by the lack of an automated information system that would allow Henry Ford Health

System to truly *manage* patient care. Pieces of an information system are in place that have allowed HFHS to accumulate information about the care that is provided, but they do not constitute an integrated information system. However, the system is taking steps likely to improve this situation in the near future. For example, a patient care information system is part of a change to creating primary care physician panels. Two other important initiatives are the Medical Information Management System and the Corporate Data Store. HFHS is designing the Medical Information Management System to integrate existing clinical and patient data systems through a common interface, allowing providers to access information about any patient's care at any time. Such a system would reduce information system redundancy and allow monitoring of patterns of care.

The Corporate Data Store is being developed as a data base integrating clinical utilization with financial and demographic data. The Corporate Data Store was conceived as a foundation for system-level quality improvement efforts, resource allocation planning, and epidemiological assessment. These data will also facilitate health services research, clinical effectiveness research, development of clinical guidelines, and cost-effectiveness studies.

A final system-level barrier to clinical integration is embedded in the Health Alliance Plan, HFHS's primary financing vehicle. The plan is structured to charge the capitated provider units when they use each other. This might unintentionally undermine clinical integration efforts.

Keys to Success at HFHS

How did the Henry Ford Health System achieve its clinical integration successes in the face of these significant obstacles? Three factors have been primarily responsible for overcoming the barriers to clinical integration: strong leadership from top management, the high quality of the system's employees, and a system culture highly compatible with the clinical integration approach.

Leadership for clinical integration was strong and originated at the top of the system, with the system CEO exhibiting a high level of commitment to clinical integration. This has been reinforced by the HFHS Corporate Quality Committee, whose monthly meetings the CEO chairs, and by the Board of Trustees Quality Committee, one of the most vital system-level board committees. By and large, the HFHS leadership is sending the right message through its pronouncements on clinical integration. While the support of top management is never a sufficient condition for successful clinical integration, it is almost always a necessary one.

HFHS is also characterized by a highly talented pool of employees, people willing to take risks and approach issues from different perspectives. Innovative projects are under way at all levels throughout the organization. People encountering a problem or issue automatically go to work to resolve it, without feeling the need to get permission or go through official channels higher up in the organization. As noted earlier, the only drawback is that these types of innovations are not always disseminated throughout the system as well as they should be.

Finally, the HFHS culture promotes self-criticism and open discussion of barriers. Issues are put on the table and dealt with, and then the process moves on. This emphasis on openness and group problem solving is highly conducive to effective clinical integration.

Lessons from the HFHS Experience

A number of lessons can be drawn from the HFHS experience with clinical integration. First, the system was right to make performance measurement an ongoing focus of its efforts. Without meaningful measurement of results, clinical integration can become an ineffective exercise, consuming organizational resources without producing tangible outcomes or opportunities for continuous improvement. On a related point, HFHS's experience—like that of several other systems in the study—points to the critical importance of well-developed information systems to support performance measurement activities.

Second, the HFHS case demonstrates the need for ongoing systemwide communication about clinical integration. Communication becomes especially crucial in systems such as HFHS that are attempting to decentralize or regionalize their planning and operations. While regionalizing may have many benefits for the system overall, HFHS may need to increase its efforts to assure dissemination of clinical integration practices and success stories throughout the system.

A third lesson from HFHS is the critical role of physicians in the clinical integration process. For successful clinical integration, systems must find ways to unify physicians behind the effort and to develop a core of physician advocates of integration.

A final lesson from HFHS is the important influence of system culture on clinical integration. In some of the systems under study, culture proved to be a barrier to clinical integration efforts. HFHS, by contrast, provides a positive example of how an open, problem-solving group culture can serve as a foundation for integration activities. Within such a culture, appropriate resources and staff support are key.

Future Directions at HFHS

As Henry Ford Health System moves into the future, it will need to look more closely at several issues related to clinical integration. These include the following:

- Determining what components are required to manage a population across a continuum of care and how these components should be organized

- Resolving the myriad physician-related challenges confronting the system, including nonaligned incentives among diverse provider groups—possible solutions might include creating an umbrella organization, with leadership from all groups, that would unite the various provider groups

- Continuing to develop information systems with an eye toward support of clinical integration activities, a process that is already under way

- Determining the most appropriate management structure for the system, given the growing emphasis on regionalization and the decision to pursue a nonowned network structure

Mercy Health Services

Mercy Health Services (MHS) represents an excellent example of what can be accomplished by a system in a relatively short time period when clinical integration becomes a real focus for system planning and activity. Clinical integration efforts at MHS were identified as a system priority and subsequently directed by a task force of representatives from throughout the system. This group developed a vision statement, work plan, clinical integration glossary, and structure of clinical integration work groups to implement integration activities at the system level. The task force also identified a set of priority clinical areas for integration efforts based on Medicare diagnosis-related groups (DRGs) profitability analysis and other data. One of the greatest strengths of Mercy's clinical integration work was the use of systemwide educational forums designed to bring employees up to speed on the rationale and core concepts of clinical integration.

Progress Toward Clinical Integration

Efforts to improve clinical integration at MHS were spearheaded by the Clinical Integration Task Force. The task force was one of a selected set of priorities identified by system leadership for immediate action. The task force was charged with enhancing clinical integration to help MHS provide appropriate, effective clinical care and improve outcomes. Membership on the task force was drawn from throughout the system, including executives and clinicians from the system's community health care systems (CHCSs) and other subsidiaries.

Major accomplishments of the clinical integration effort at MHS included the following:

- Development of a vision statement for clinical integration activities

- Design of a clinical integration work plan

- Production of a clinical integration glossary

- Selection of priority DRGs/clinical areas for initial focus of clinical integration efforts

- Systemwide educational efforts

- Formation of clinical integration work groups

Both the vision statement and the clinical integration glossary were developed to increase the understanding of clinical integration throughout MHS. The vision states the following:

MHS Clinical Integration assures a coordinated system of appropriate, effective clinical care which:
- includes a seamless continuum of services in which care is provided in the most appropriate setting;
- improves community health status;
- involves caregivers from all disciplines;
- supports collaborative practice among clinicians, within and between CHCSs.

The glossary contains detailed definitions of sixty-five commonly used terms related to clinical integration. A clinical integration resources guide was also developed, listing published sources of information on clinical integration, algorithms, critical pathways, practice guidelines and protocols, outcomes management, and specific clinical practice areas.

In order to decide on priority areas for the clinical integration effort, the task force considered Medicare profitability analysis data from fiscal year 1992, results of a CEO survey, and potential impacts on cost and quality of implementing clinical integration in various clinical areas. The profitability analysis data was also disseminated throughout the system to call attention to the need for clinical integration efforts. The seven priority areas identified by the task force were coronary artery disease, heart failure and shock, stroke, pneumonia, joint replacement, psychosis, and ventilator management. Individual community health care systems within MHS helped to identify the seven priority areas and then decided which priority areas to target at the local system level.

The task force increased systemwide learning of clinical care process innovations through educational forums attended by hundreds of clinicians and administrators from throughout MHS. Resources such as critical pathways and algorithms were disseminated to the individual community health care systems. The task force also formed three work groups to lend additional support to clinical integration activities. The Forums Work Group was charged with addressing variations in practice patterns and sharing approaches to clinical integration. The Clinical Consulting Teams Work Group was formed to design the methodology for clinical integration care processes and to identify and prepare consulting team members. The Tools and Resources Work Group was set up to identify existing and needed tools and resources for clinical integration, including data resources.

After completing the activities described above, the task force developed a second-generation work plan to carry clinical integration efforts forward into the future, with primary focus on two main strategies: (1) maximizing the appropriate use of resources across MHS and within the community health care system (CHCS) through efficient, effective care and movement of patients throughout the system; and (2) supporting local CHCSs to achieve improved quality and financial performance in key clinical areas, improving clinical integration across all settings in the CHCSs. Priority work groups for the second-generation work plan were established to examine case/care management, clinical integration data, clinical integration progress, outcomes measurement, and clinical integration education.

Obstacles to Integration

Mercy Health Services had to overcome many significant barriers in its attempt to achieve greater clinical integration within the system. Some of the most daunting obstacles in the path to clinical integration included an insufficient base of physician integration, insufficient physician leadership, and the dispersed geography and large size of the system, which made effective intrasystem communication difficult. Other obstacles included budgeting policies and practices that were not based on cross-unit clinical service lines, underdeveloped information systems, and nonrelational data systems. Many of these difficulties were not entirely overcome, but instead represent continuing challenges for the system.

In addition, in most of Mercy's markets there is a relatively low level of capitation and managed care penetration, thus removing some of the incentive for achieving clinical integration. There was also the need for greater cooperation among various components of the system. For example, case managers for Mercy Health Plans—the system's managed care arm—were not consistently allowed access to medical records and other critical information about their enrollees within the system. Each facility seemed to have its own policy regarding the degree of information sharing it would allow with Mercy Health Plans. Also, each community health care system had its own manner of interaction with Amicare, Mercy's home care subsidiary.

A final significant barrier to clinical integration at MHS was the system culture, which was described as defender-like and with a reluctance to use data. Some informants within the system felt the culture of MHS resulted in slow decision making and a lack of clear-cut direction to units within the system. There was also a perception that CQI was not being used to its full potential, partly because of financial pressures but also because of lack of accountability for implementation and lack of emphasis on CQI by system leaders. Some interviewees also noted the need to develop a greater level of trust between hospitals and physicians and between those involved in inpatient and outpatient settings.

Keys to Success at MHS

Despite these obstacles, MHS achieved impressive successes in the area of clinical integration. These successes were made possible, in large part, by the strong leadership provided by the Clinical Integration Task Force, with its representation from various components of the system and its focus on improving communication and coordination within the clinical integration process. Additional leadership came from the Office of Professional and Physician Services, which played an important role in promoting information sharing through forums and conferences.

MHS created a number of valuable opportunities for intrasystem communication. One example was a clinical integration conference that brought together all the cardiovascular leaders from throughout the system. Participants shared information on what is done in the various regions, discussed future strategies and better ways of handling intrasystem referrals, and identified potential areas for coordinated efforts in the future. The conference included the CEOs of most of the Michigan hospitals and at least one cardiologist and one cardiovascular surgeon from each institution.

Similar information-sharing efforts occurred among Mercy's behavioral medicine professionals, who met on a bimonthly basis for a "Behavioral Medicine Think Tank." These meetings grew out of a perceived need to develop a carve-out behavioral services product for payers. The group addressed ways to better coordinate care across the system and to appropriately and consistently measure the outcomes of their services. Similarly, an annual fall conference for nursing and allied health services within MHS created cross-system communication opportunities, although this conference tended to be focused primarily on acute care issues.

Individual institutions and community health care systems within MHS implemented additional changes to foster greater clinical integration. At St. Joseph's Mercy Hospital, Pontiac, a vice president for care process integration was assigned to coordinate clinical integration in the region. Two clinical administrators and two patient care coordinators at the institution reported directly to this newly created position. This hospital also created four service lines—each with its own service line manager—in primary care, specialty areas, geriatrics, and behavioral medicine. Service line managers were charged with coordinating and marketing all the needed care to their respective constituencies.

A number of changes were introduced to enhance clinical integration in the McAuley Health System (Ann Arbor, Michigan). A plan was developed to allow McAuley physicians to share in the savings brought about by clinical integration efforts. This arrangement appeared to be one promising way to build trust between the physicians and the system and to increase physicians' incentives for supporting integration activities. Other important innovations at McAuley included the development of the Academic Internal Medicine (AIM) unit at St. Joseph's Hospital in Ann Arbor, which used an interdisciplinary team approach to focus on improving care for "frequent flyers," high-risk patients with frequent readmissions to the hospital (some to the point of spending more than half of the year as inpatients). The team consisted of staff dedicated to the unit, including attending physicians, residents, nurses, a social worker, a pharmacist, a chemical dependency worker, and a home care coordinator.

The team worked cooperatively to coordinate care within the unit, and appropriate personnel also followed the patients in outpatient clinic settings. The unit developed protocols of treatment for particularly difficult patients so that when these patients appeared in the emergency room, their course of care had already been mapped out. The patients actually brought these care protocols with them to the ER. One crucial feature of the AIM unit was that virtually all physicians working on the unit worked for the Department of Internal Medicine. There were few private practitioners caring for patients on this unit. The various innovations employed by this unit significantly reduced length of stay and cost per case to the point that the unit had the lowest average on these two measures in the entire hospital.

Lessons from the MHS Experience

Important lessons can be gleaned from MHS's clinical integration efforts. First, we see the need to identify clinical integration as a systemwide priority and consequently communicate this priority to the entire system. Mercy's experience demonstrates the paramount importance of communication and information sharing within systems as a way to "grease the wheels" of clinical integration. Effective intrasystem communication is especially crucial (and also more difficult) for systems like MHS that are large and geographically dispersed.

Mercy's experience also points to the need for clear, strategic direction guiding clinical integration efforts. The Clinical Integration Task Force's identification of priority areas was a good starting point, but there is the need to flesh out the clinical integration plan, to disseminate it throughout the system, and to clarify the expectations flowing from the plan.

It is difficult to overemphasize the importance of strong leadership and a supportive system culture for achieving clinical integration. Although Mercy enjoyed some significant successes, the system's progress toward clinical integration might have been faster and smoother with even stronger leadership and a culture fostering innovation and change. Mercy's short-term orientation and somewhat defender-like culture in all likelihood slowed down clinical integration in many subtle ways that are difficult to quantify. Mercy's example demonstrates that system leaders need to stress the importance of the CQI philosophy frequently and in a wide range of forums to keep CQI as a cornerstone of clinical integration.

The Mercy example also suggests the importance of making sure that all components of a system are working together in a coordinated fashion toward the goal of clinical integration. In Mercy's case, it was troubling to see that the system's own home health service (Amicare) was not consistently used by other units within the system, and also that case managers for the managed care subsidiary (Mercy Health Plans) had difficulty accessing the records of some enrollees who received care in the system. At a more general level, reports of tensions between physicians and the system and between inpatient and outpatient components of the system suggest the continuing challenges to be faced.

Facing the Future

In its second-generation work plan, the Clinical Integration Task Force laid out several tactics to advance clinical integration efforts. These tactics included the following:

- Communicating information about cost, quality, anticipated service needs, and impact of volume

- Identifying opportunities for enhancing patient referrals across MHS community health care systems, by locating existing areas of clinical excellence and piloting new referral models

- Developing a process for monitoring and evaluating progress toward clinical integration in the seven clinical priority areas

- Providing support for clinical practice innovation

- Developing common approaches to outcome measurement

- Identifying and developing infrastructure elements needed to achieve clinical integration, including a case management system, a clinical information system, a longitudinal patient care record, and a preferred drug approach and formulary

Successful implementation of these tactics would undoubtedly strengthen clinical integration within MHS.

At a more general level, MHS needs to more clearly determine its focus as a system. Will its focus be at the level of the community health care systems, at the level of the regions served, or at the level of the system as a whole? This is an important question, as its answer will dictate how clinical integration activities are carried out.

Another area for possible consideration is Mercy's relationships with its physicians, especially in terms of the role physicians are expected to play in the system. MHS needs to become a more physician-centered organization and accelerate physician involvement in clinical integration and other important initiatives. Toward this end, MHS would benefit from a formal physician leadership development program. Existing programs around the country could serve as models, or could be used to train Mercy physicians, in order to increase the number of physicians who can play significant roles in clinical integration. MHS also should accelerate its development of physician group practices.

MHS should consider realignment of incentives and organizational structures within the system to anticipate major changes in the health care environment and to promote integration efforts. In other words, MHS—like all systems striving for clinical integration—should move toward rewarding people for how well the system or region does rather than for the performance of individual units within the system. This kind of realignment encourages people to make the changes that will improve system performance as a whole, even when the bottom line of individual units may be adversely affected. More broadly, MHS should consider "biting the bullet"; that is, being willing to take some short-run losses in order to realign the organization for the future and thereby promote long-run gain. For example, Mercy might experiment by having one of its regions reorganize *as if* payment in that region were 100 percent capitated.

In the area of planning, MHS is like many systems in its efforts to move from institution-based to population-based approaches. MHS should focus on developing a Community Health Status Needs Assessment, a potentially valuable tool for population-based planning. Each community health care system within MHS should plan and organize its services based on the needs of the population and the associated employers and payers of care in the area. Greater emphasis must be placed on the primary care needs of the population and on developing the associated organization of physicians, nurses, and other health professionals to meet those needs. Hospital-focused planning must be de-emphasized.

Finally, MHS needs to make further progress toward involving representatives from the full continuum of care, rather than from only the hospitals, in the system's clinical integration efforts. While hospital-based clinical care often represents a logical starting point for integration efforts, true clinical integration requires the participation of all levels of caregiving. All interested parties should be included in clinical integration efforts from the beginning of planning activities, even if the initial efforts do not involve the complete continuum of care. MHS needs to ensure that outpatient interests are adequately represented in these efforts. Without this kind of broad-based participation, clinical integration runs the risk of being perceived as just another hospital quality project. More generally, Mercy Health Services will need to ensure that both inpatient and outpatient perspectives are represented and given adequate voice in top management discussions regarding the direction of the system.

UniHealth

UniHealth, an organized delivery system consisting of Care America Health Plan, seven hospitals, seven medical groups, and CliniShare home health services, is strategically committed to improving performance through comprehensive outcomes measurement and continuous quality improvement. These efforts began in a systematic way in 1989. By investigating "best practices key levers," factors strongly linked to significant process improvement are discovered, validated, and disseminated systemwide, expediting the diffusion of innovations with proven process improvement potential. In 1993, clinical case management, an activity that had emerged in several UniHealth hospitals, was identified as a key lever associated with reduced length of stay and cost per case for congestive heart failure (CHF) and angina patients at UniHealth's California Hospital Medical Center (CHMC). The clinical case managers are registered nurses, who work directly with physicians, nurses, and other caregivers to coordinate comprehensive patient care plans, expedite achievement of target outcomes, monitor and guide patient progress, and maximize the patient and family's self-care potential. To date, use of clinical case managers at CHMC has resulted in significant reductions in length of stay and estimated savings of over $2.5 million. Concurrently, Uni-Health's Glendale Memorial Hospital was conducting a unit-based "micro management" care coordination project for a group of congestive heart failure patients. They reported length of stay and cost reductions of over $1,000 per case, as well as increased patient satisfaction validated through outcomes measures.

California Hospital Medical Center clinical case managers (CCMs) provide an example of how the process works. The CCMs focused on clinical service integration and efficiency within and between UniHealth and non-UniHealth entities. Upon admission, the CCM reviewed the patient's history and current status, and sought previous records and test results, avoiding redundancy and linking the current episode with relevant past tests, treatment, and ongoing care. At discharge, the CCM bridged communication with the primary care physician and community health agencies. Again, the process resulted in significant reductions in costs, length of stay, and readmissions.

Based on the above results, the Patient Care Leadership Team of affiliate Patient Care Vice Presidents proposed a systemwide initiative in which staff would be recruited for new strategic CCM positions and provided competency-driven role development education. Goals of this initiative were to optimize coordination of patient care, reduce clinical process variation, optimize clinical process effectiveness and appropriateness, enhance quality and outcomes, reduce cost per case through increased efficiency, and ensure the adoption of best practices. UniHealth's significant investment in the development and delivery of the CCM course was derived from knowledge that clinical competency, prerequisite to RN work assignments in the CCM role, is acquired through post-licensure continuing education and work experience. RNs with this expertise are in short supply in the UniHealth System and across southern California in general.

The Clinical Case Management Curriculum

The UniHealth Clinical Case Management curriculum consists of nine instructional modules geared to practicing RNs or other professionals in contemporary health care delivery. Based on principles of adult learning and "distance education," the UniHealth CCM modules combine workshop-based instruction, clinical experiences, and highly self-directed study. While the program is specifically designed for prospective clinical case managers, portions of the curriculum may be relevant to other staff and may be offered to a broader audience as needed.

The modules in the Clinical Case Management curriculum are as follows:

Module 1   Introduction to Clinical Case Management

Module 2   Collaborative Interdisciplinary Relationships

Module 3   Selection and Management of Target Populations

Module 4   Development and Implementation of Clinical Paths

Module 5   Evaluation of Clinical Process Variance and Patient Outcomes

Module 6   Clinical Case Management Outcomes Processes as Quality Control and Improvement Strategies

Module 7   Optimization of Patient/Family Outcomes Through Self-Care

Module 8   Leadership for Organizational Change and Innovation

Module 9   Clinical Case Management Across the Continuum

Because the modules reflect to some extent the clinical case management process, taking the modules in sequence is ideal. However, the last four modules may be taken in any sequence. The nine modules in the Clinical Case Management curriculum are designed to be presented over a sixteen-week period, generally introducing a new module every two weeks. Learners receive each module syllabus two to four weeks in advance of each scheduled workshop.

Module 1, Introduction to Clinical Case Management, provides an overview of the concepts underpinning the entire curriculum and must be taken first. With the successful completion of Modules 1 and 2, the participant is encouraged to integrate role-specific clinical experiences that parallel the case management process.

Module 9 provides an overview of the continuum of care process and of the clinical case manager role as a bridge from acute care to ambulatory care. The participants are encouraged to implement strategies needed to resolve problems that occur across the continuum through ambulatory services. A partial content outline for Module 9 is presented below as an illustration of the program.

I. Demand for care coordination/clinical case management across the care continuum
   A. Role of community-based care in the health care continuum
      1. Current
      2. Anticipated
   C. Application of clinical case management in the community setting
      1. Driving forces
         a. Economic
         b. Sociopolitical
         c. Technological
      2. Incentives of payers and providers
      3. Challenge of integration
      4. High priority of continuum of care
      5. Leadership by physicians
      6. Benefits management
      7. Optimization of functional health status
   D. Inpatient versus outpatient clinical case management
      1. Similarities
      2. Differences
      3. Integration
II. Coordination of care across the continuum
   D. Models of community-based case management
      1. Disease management model

2. Symptom management model

3. Utilization review models

F. Algorithms, pathways, guidelines, and education

1. Goal planning

2. Service integration

3. Quality care cycle

4. Comprehensive health education

5. Comprehensive interview and evaluation

6. Provider evaluation

G. Clinical case manager support systems

1. Management systems

2. Quality management systems

3. Information management systems

4. Financial systems

III. Collaboration and integration of care across the continuum

C. Communication and feedback strategies

1. Building trust among providers

2. Expanding walls concept

3. Feedback mechanisms

D. Integrated systems

1. Definitions

2. Emerging CCM role implications

E. Tools for enhancing collaboration, integration, and quality outcomes management

1. Discharge plans

2. Clinical practice guidelines

3. Practice parameters

4. Clinical paths

5. CareMap™

IV. Stabilizing patients in home settings

B. Identification of high risk issues

1. Acute clinical conditions

2. Chronic clinical conditions

3. High utilization of services

4. Health behaviors and compliance

5. Medication utilization

6. Falls

7. Skin integrity

8. Nutrition

C. Patient/family participation in home health care

1. Issues

2. Strategies

Barriers and Challenges

The greatest challenge to implementing the UniHealth CCM Role Development Program was the inherent diversity of the staff and of the different hospitals involved. Given the variety of clinical and strategic initiatives characteristic of UniHealth affiliate hospitals, the systemwide CCM education program was challenged to provide training that recognized and incorporated variation in how the role was implemented. Likewise, the organizational climates in which the graduate CCMs were expected to perform their roles varied in their readiness to support the CCM. Because the term *case manager* had been broadly and loosely used to define a range of activities including utilization review, discharge planning, and clinical care coordination, it was critical to the success of the project to define the term *clinical case manager* and clarify the role to prevent confusion and conflict. Physicians and other staff differed in their understanding of the role and in their readiness to collaborate.

A related challenge has been to develop a systemwide approach to clinical pathway variance analysis. In the meantime, the ability of the CCMs to use and conduct such analysis varies greatly by hospital.

The new CCMs are also challenged to integrate their services and to link payers and home health case managers in order to optimally coordinate care. CCMs must exert leadership among their peers and colleagues and consistently communicate complex information that addresses all of the patients' needs. The emphasis must continually be on communication and teamwork.

Finally, managed care demands CCM expertise in patient, family, and caregiver education, outcomes measurement, payer finance/utilization, and data analysis and presentation. While these concepts are covered in the UniHealth CCM curriculum, CCMs have requested quarterly matrix team meetings that help them develop skills in these key and related areas. Investing in basic role development supports "entry into practice" for case managers and analyzes the challenge of ongoing role development.

Major Facilitators and Lessons

The office of the president, the chief medical officer, and the Patient Care Leadership Team (PCLT) have been essential to the success of the CCM program. Despite a culture of diversity, UniHealth affiliates have been clearly committed to the strategic potential of the CCM. It is important to note that the Patient Care Leadership Team collaborated in identifying the core competencies for role development and participated in developing and refining the CCM curriculum. The first forty-eight CCMs to attend the course were hand picked by the affiliate patient care executives (PCEs); their assignments and preliminary clinical outcomes are being closely monitored by the PCLT.

The UniHealth CCM program benefited from expertise within UniHealth and from external consultation. In retrospect, the staff support and effort required to develop and implement the CCM training program was underestimated. Despite the service of a consulting instructional designer, the scope of the nine-module project, the review and refinement of the developing instructional materials, the selection of supplemental journal literature and texts, and the delivery of nine conference-type workshops all required significant professional and clerical staff support.

The project coordinator, a doctoral-level nurse with previously established faculty credentials at a regional university, arranged for UniHealth employees who completed the CCM program to receive academic extension credit. Several students reported that participation in the CCM course renewed their interest in higher education.

Because they enjoyed the challenges of learning, experienced success, and earned academic credit, they were motivated to pursue
new educational goals.

The CCM workshops also created a mutually supportive network
of peers that encouraged learning and early role development. "Sea-
soned" CCMs have served as instructors in the second CCM course
and have mentored new CCMs. In particular, the integration of home
health staff with their acute care peers has been beneficial.

As the role of the hospital-based CCM evolves, there will be additional opportunities to integrate case management services among
the system's medical groups, hospitals, and home health agencies.

Ongoing evaluation of the impact of the CCM role is taking
place. Structured interviews with CCMs, key physicians, and clinical supervisors suggest that the role is effective in enhancing the
coordination and integration of acute care services. Several physicians have reported that the CCM makes them more aware of
practice variation among their colleagues and of ways to reduce
unnecessary variation. UniHealth is also in the midst of examining
risk-adjusted case mix data and collecting prospective patient satisfaction data that will quantify outcomes for the implementation of
the CCM role in terms of length of stay, readmission, cost per case,
and customer satisfaction. This will be particularly important in managing the increased incidence and prevalence of chronic illness in
a managed care environment.

Future Strategies and Issues

To succeed in its reengineering efforts, UniHealth must continue its
innovative work force cross-training and career development initiatives.

To date, forty-eight staff members have completed the UniHealth
CCM curriculum, representing six of the seven UniHealth hospitals
and CliniShare, UniHealth's home health entity. Evaluation of the
impact of the first cohort of thirteen new CCMs on outcomes measures is in progress. Qualitative internal benchmark data will be integrated with qualitative data gleaned from interviews with practicing

UniHealth CCMs, physicians, and administrators. Upon completion of the first CCM evaluation, UniHealth expects to better understand what role CCMs will play in integration efforts, what the barriers and facilitators are to optimal role performance, and what direction future training should take.

Future Issues

As we have stated previously, clinical integration is difficult, life-long work. Many of the issues raised in this chapter will continue to occupy systems' attention for years to come. But three issues particularly stand out. These are the challenges of managing an increasing number of Americans with chronic illness; of adjusting care processes to incorporate new technologies, treatments, and prevention practices; and of coping with "carve out" benefits and associated financing.

The Growth of Chronic Illness

The challenges of chronic illness are directly associated with the aging of the population, particularly with individuals eighty-five and older. Since 1980 there has been a 22 percent increase in the percentage of the population sixty-five years and older, and this group is expected to more than double in size between 1990 and 2030 (Kane, 1994, pp. 9–10). The eighty-five–plus group will triple in size between 1990 and 2030. The health care system, and hospitals in particular, are ill equipped to deal with this growth, as evidenced by a recent survey indicating that only 5 percent of responding hospitals felt they were "highly ready" to deal with the needs of the elderly population and only 43 percent believed they were moderately ready (Kane and others, 1994). To put it briefly: "How do integrated health care organizations move from being 'brick and mortar' continuums of care to coordinated-care systems that truly manage patient care and guide patients along clinical pathways that are appropriate to the level and acuity needs of the patient?" (Kane, 1994, p. 11).

One of the biggest challenges in dealing with the multiple chronic illnesses of an aging society may lie in changing even experts' views of the acute care hospital as the hub for delivering and coordinating such care (Kane, 1994). Given that hospitals are no longer the hub of the overall delivery system, it would seem a giant backward step to charge them with central responsibility for coordinating care for those with multiple chronic illnesses. It is not surprising that the majority of hospitals do not feel that they are ready to deal with the challenge. The more relevant question is whether one should even expect it of them. We think the target is misplaced.

Although there will always be an acute care component to managing most chronic illnesses, we believe the "organizer" of the continuum of care for patients suffering from multiple chronic illnesses will be the home health care agency working jointly with the patient's personal physician. For example, the leading chronic health conditions of older populations are arthritis, hypertension, hearing impairment, and heart disease—all of which can be most effectively managed on an outpatient, primary care, home health care basis. As evidence of this, the number of Medicare enrollees using home care has risen fivefold over the past fifteen years, and three out of four home care users are Medicare enrollees (Hing, 1994).

Thus, a major challenge for organized delivery systems in achieving greater levels of clinical integration for managing the care of patients with chronic illnesses is to organize the continuum of care around home health and primary care rather than around acute inpatient care. In doing so, many study systems and others around the country (Coile, 1995) have learned that such patients cannot be managed with individual protocols but rather require case management approaches; that because of the demands created by multiple chronic illness, the case management approach must extend broadly across many delivery settings and types of providers; that *continuous* monitoring is required, placing unique demands on clinical information systems; and that physicians and other health care professionals caring for chronically ill patients require additional multidisciplinary training in geriatrics in order to adequately meet the needs of this segment of the population. Most of the study systems do not see their hospitals playing a dominant role in this regard. Rather, the opposite appears to be the case. That is, the extent to which hospital resources are required to treat the chronically ill represents a *failure* on the part of the rest of the system to achieve appropriate levels of continuity of care and clinical integration to effectively manage the chronically ill.

Technology

New technologies, treatments, and disease prevention breakthroughs will always disrupt current approaches to caring for patients. Thus what appears to be clinically integrated today may not be tomorrow. Systems must be open to these new developments and flexible in incorporating those that are likely to add value for patients. The Community Clinical Oncology Program (CCOP), designed to increase community participation in National Cancer Institute–approved clinical trials, represents a prototype example (Kaluzny and others, 1996). We believe that new technologies, treatments, and disease prevention innovations all point in the same direction—to more care delivered in outpatient settings, in the patient's home, in physician offices, and in the workplace. A premium will be placed on cost-reducing technologies that increase longevity and quality of life. New drug therapies, biotechnology advances, gene therapy, and related developments are examples of this trend and are discussed further in Chapter Eight.

One implication of this trend is that clinical integration and continuum of care efforts that are now largely focused around acute inpatient episodes will need to expand and be refocused around a much broader continuum of care. The second implication is that clinical integration will need to shift from the current dominant practice of using protocols, pathways, and case management approaches *after* the patient has developed a problem to an *anticipatory* mode of *planning in advance* for the disease and illnesses the patient will likely develop in a world of "predict and prevent" technology. It is not unreasonable to expect that in the near future, the health and social services that individuals will need throughout their lifetime will be reasonably predictable shortly after their birth.

Carve Outs

There is a current fascination with carve out benefits and programs in such areas as mental health, substance abuse, long-term care, pharmaceuticals, and even in such areas as cardiovascular and cancer care. While one can understand the reasons for these developments, it is important to consider whether they impede the ability to achieve a more clinically integrated continuum of care for patients. Carve outs simply perpetuate and, indeed, accelerate the fragmentation and suboptimization of care that currently exists. Most patients and their families experience health problems that go beyond a specialized need of the moment. Providers and systems that hold contracts for one carve out service may not hold contracts for another, causing patients to deal with multiple provider entities and systems. The challenge of transferring medical records and information and monitoring the patients' overall health status are enormous. The problems caused by carve outs are likely to grow with the increasing numbers of older patients with multiple chronic illnesses. Under carve out benefits and financing, these patients will figuratively (and, perhaps, occasionally literally) be "carved out" among multiple providers and systems, defeating all of the objectives of more clinically integrated holistic care. Eliminating carve out benefits and financing will require the political leadership of system management and governance as well as leadership from caregivers. Some of the additional managerial and governance challenges to creating organized delivery systems are discussed in Chapter Seven.

Governance and Management
Constructing a Solid Foundation

To thrive, even survive, in today's new marketplace,
your health care organization must create a new
infrastructure. The framework on which your
organization will be built must be flexible, inclusive,
and farsighted.

J. R. Griffith, *"The Infrastructure*
of Integrated Delivery Systems," 1995, p. 12.

Today, most health care organizations around the country are
pursuing a variety of strategies, all in the name of integration.
"They are experimenting to find out what works and what doesn't
work. It's like the search for the Holy Grail. . . . Everyone believes
integration is the way to go, but no one can point to any one system that is all the way there" (Bartling, 1995, p. 10). As did our
study participants, many systems focus first on the concepts described earlier: integrating various nonclinical functions (for example, human resources, planning, finance, managed care); aligning
more closely with key physicians in the marketplace (that is, physician-system integration); and pursuing the ultimate of integration
efforts—clinical integration. All of these efforts are necessary if an
organization is to become a delivery system that can coordinate a
continuum of services for a defined population. However, none of

these integration efforts will succeed in the long term unless a system's governance and management structures are aligned with and actively supportive of these efforts.

As described in Chapter Three, building an organized delivery system (ODS) is like building a home overlooking a canyon. One must begin by installing strong pillars in bedrock to create the underpinnings for a solid foundation. "Without a strong foundation, even the most impressive home is in peril. The same is true for organized delivery systems" (Griffith, 1995, p. 12). For an ODS, these pillars (its vision, culture, strategy, and leadership) are either strengthened or weakened by a system's governance and management. Indeed, an *effective* governance and management structure will create a clear vision for the organization, foster a culture supportive of that vision, enable the organization to implement its strategies, and provide the leadership necessary to guide ongoing change and ensure accountability to multiple stakeholders— patients, payers, regulators, the community, and others.

Unfortunately, no standard, "off the shelf" governance or management structures (or models) are universally applicable to all organized delivery systems. When you've seen one organized delivery system, you've seen one organized delivery system. Furthermore, the interdependent, collaborative nature of an ODS also "limits the extent to which existing governance forms employed by stand-alone institutions or multi-hospital systems can be merely 'brought forward' or 'carried over'" (Pointer, Alexander, and Zuckerman, 1995, p. 4) to an ODS. Consequently, a significant challenge organizations will face on their integration journey will be in designing the "right" governance and management model for their specific system (and market) at a given point in time.

The optimal ODS governance and management structure must be sensitive to the organization's unique history, culture, and current structure (stage of evolution), as well as responsive to the specific characteristics of its market, including its likely speed of transformation. Before an organization can create a structure that addresses its unique situation, it will have to reexamine the "theory of the business," based on the basic assumptions upon which the organization has been built (Drucker, 1994). As noted in Chapters One and Two, those organizations that continue to operate under the old theory, where the hospital is the center of the delivery system, will fail. The organization must make new assumptions about the environment, societal expectations, the market, the customer, and technology. It must also make new assumptions about its specific mission and the core competencies and capabilities needed to achieve the mission. These assumptions must fit reality, and they must be consistent with each other, understood by all involved, and tested continuously.

Once these fundamental issues and future parameters have been defined, the organization must design governance and management structures that will facilitate the development and performance of a truly integrated company. To date, no clear approach has been adopted consistently by the more progressive integrated delivery systems around the country. Instead, systems are experimenting with every conceivable combination and permutation of governance and management structures. As a starting point, many systems are exploring adaptations of models that seemed to work for traditional multihospital systems. Three of the more common governance structures under review include (1) the parent holding company, characterized by a systemwide corporate governing board and separate boards at the operating-unit level; (2) the modified parent holding company, characterized by one systemwide governing board with advisory boards substituted for governing boards at the operating-unit level; and (3) the corporate model, characterized by one systemwide governing board with no local governing or advisory boards (Morlock and Alexander, 1986). Although none of these models are ideal, organizations can piece together various elements of the different models to create structures suitable to their current needs.

As the above models suggest, traditional multihospital systems have been focused on governance models in which the assets of the facilities are controlled and owned through a common parent structure or a singular corporate model. These models have worked relatively well for horizontal integration, in which independent hospitals have combined with other hospitals to form systems. However, as discussed in Chapter Three, the success of an organized delivery system will be characterized by the degree to which it creates a seamless continuum of care that links organizations at different stages of the health care delivery process.

To select the preferred governance model available, an organization must decide how it will organize along four key dimensions: control, structure, functioning, and composition.

- *Control.*   First and foremost, an organization must determine whether or not it will be governed by a *centralized* board (the corporate model) or a *decentralized* board (either the parent holding company or modified parent holding company model).

- *Structure.*   If the organization adopts a decentralized structure, it will need to clarify how its "subordinate" boards should be utilized—should a subordinate board be created for each operating unit, each region (if regions are necessary), or each group of operating units (for example, a subordinate board over the system's hospitals, long-term care facilities, medical groups, and so forth)? Some systems find that the most suitable structure requires a combination of these various options (for example, a board for each operating unit, which reports to a regional board, which then reports to the system board).

- *Functioning.*   A system that has chosen to organize around multiple boards must clearly delineate the powers and authorities vested at each board level. Another option would be to have one "true" governing body at the system level and "advisory boards" at the institutional and/or regional levels.

- *Composition.*   The organization must determine whether the overall system of governance will be representative or nonrepresentative. In representative boards, members are selected based on their relationship to a particular operating unit; with a nonrepresentative approach, elected members have no relationship to various components of the system. For example, a representative system would be one that provides each operating unit with a seat on the parent board. The disadvantage of this type of system, however, would be that as the system grows the board will also grow and it may reach an unmanageable size. Furthermore, representative governance structures tend to impede systemness, because each board member often focuses on furthering the interests of his or her particular institution rather than striving to improve the position of the system overall. Likewise, organizations must also make a conscious effort to recruit board members with specific skill sets to serve on the board of an integrated delivery system (Pointer, Alexander and Zuckerman, 1995).

What we have learned from the study systems suggests that creating a continuum of care is essential. This effort in turn drives systems to adopt a vertical, rather than horizontal, integration strategy—important, based on the study findings, because a vertical integration strategy does not require that all parts of the system be owned and controlled by the same parent. This finding is particularly helpful in creating relationships between physicians and purchasers. Physicians, for a variety of reasons, may lose some of their appeal in the marketplace if they are locked within a "closed system." One lesson from the failure of the Clinton "managed competition" health care proposal was that many Americans were not interested in selecting large closed systems that would preclude freedom of access to the provider of their choice.

Because completely closed systems are not generally accepted, a vertical integration strategy will be flawed if it predicates organizational success on common control and ownership of all parts of the system. A more appropriate implementation of the vertical integration strategy is to ensure that *virtual integration,* or what we call *behavioral* integration, occurs through implementing effective contractual relationships (Goldsmith, 1994).

The experience of the study systems also suggests that two other "V's" are important to implementing a vertical integration strategy. The first of these is that vertically integrated organizations must reflect *visual integration.* In other words, the consumer must perceive and experience the products and services produced by the organized delivery system as being seamless. As discussed in previous chapters, organized delivery systems that effectively meet the challenges of the new health care environment will have holographic qualities. When an organized delivery system behaves like a hologram, visual integration is achieved.

The second "V" can best be described as *visceral integration,* or the degree to which the partners in a vertically integrated relationship regard the system's success to be of significant importance. The partners must have an emotional and pocketbook commitment to the strategy, not merely an intellectual commitment to it. The key distinction is the ability to commit financial and human resources to the strategy so that its partners will feel pain if the system is not successful in reaching its goals. As one system executive described this level of commitment, "It is a time in which we cannot have deep pockets and short arms." System leaders must be willing to commit appropriate resources to the vertical integration strategy and then implement and manage it aggressively.

ODSs are also experimenting with management infrastructures, which they recognize must be collaborative, team based, supportive of staff empowerment, and designed to allow for systematic up-grades in the way decisions are made and people are motivated (Charns and Smith-Tewksbury, 1993; Griffith, 1995). New management teams will evolve to address issues across the system and within regions. And, while one individual may continue to manage one function, he or she will do so across multiple, integrated sites. Thus, the maturing ODS becomes an organization without walls—one whose management structure meets both internal and external (community) needs.

Finally, as stated previously, physician leaders are key to integration efforts. Consequently, no matter how organizations structure their governance and senior management functions, physician leaders must play a critical leadership role. ODSs empower system physicians by allocating board seats (with voting rights) on all significant boards within the system. Further, physicians in senior management positions serve not only in staff/support roles (for example, senior vice president for medical staff affairs) but also have increasing line authority and responsibility embodied in their positions (for example, senior executive over physician practices and ambulatory services).

Barriers and Challenges

Futurist Joel Barker has noted that it is the anticipation of what the future will look like that has allowed organizations to transform themselves prior to significant industry and market changes. This confident expectation of and preparation for a new environment has resulted in organizations finding themselves in the right place at the right time to realize ongoing success (Barker, 1992). However, in the world of health care, integrated delivery is clearly the direction in which organizations are heading, yet few seem to have successfully created a system of care that they would characterize as truly integrated. What makes this journey so difficult? From an overall management and governance perspective, we believe that five major barriers or challenges impede a system's integration efforts:

(1) historical roles and responsibilities, (2) inability to understand and internalize the new health care environment, (3) shortage of talent with the "right" skills, (4) fear of losing control, and (5) fear of failure. An organization's governance, management, and aligned physicians must respond with strong leadership if the organization is to overcome these barriers, as discussed below.

Historical Roles and Responsibilities

Shedding the weight of the past is unquestionably one of the most difficult challenges organizations will face over the next several years. All systems, structures, personnel, and reward mechanisms have been designed to support a model of care very different from that required of tomorrow's successful providers. In the past, the focus was on treating illness, caring for the individual, and filling schedules and beds by increasing visits and admissions. In this world the hospital was king, and all governance and management activities were designed to support that reign. As a result, "it is time to pay due respect to the past—perhaps even grieve over it—but then to get on with inventing and managing the new delivery systems to meet the needs of the future" (Shortell, Gillies, and others, 1993, pp. 452–453).

The new health care organization will be responsible for a very different set of activities. It must become accountable for health status and maintaining wellness; provide access to a continuum of care and services that are "value added"; deliver care in the most cost-effective manner and in the most appropriate location; manage a network of services that it likely will not own; and actively manage quality. Since the rush to integration began, most hospital-based health care delivery systems have been assembling the "right pieces" to prepare for their new responsibilities. However, their focus has been on filling in their continuums of care, through either strategic alliances or outright acquisitions, rather than on developing the necessary infrastructure to make the pieces work well together.

In particular, many systems are collapsing structures to force a "desegregation" and, they hope, an integration of their operating units. However, it is important to note that integration and deseg-regation are not the same. Integration and centralization are also very different concepts. As described above, integration requires an interactive, interdependent relationship to be formed among the various "integrated" entities. Simply aggregating a system's operat-ing units into a common reporting structure will not create a seam-less, well-coordinated health care system. These distinctions are critical and, if comprehended, will help an organization revise var-ious roles and responsibilities throughout the system to facilitate and support the desired change.

In the past, governing bodies were dominated by hospital issues, hospital people, and an interest in continuing to spend resources on the creation of a facility-rich empire. Board structures generally were decentralized and cumbersome, often reflecting a variation of the holding-company model described earlier. Each operating unit gen-erally had its own board, and as long as that unit performed within the agreed-upon financial parameters and did not pursue activities that conflicted with the mission, the board was free to pursue what-ever strategy it chose for its market. However, as organizations reor-ganize to become more integrated, governance can no longer be an "afterthought. . . . Issues of governance are pivotal and left unat-tended may serve as barriers to, rather than facilitators of, successful system integration and success" (Pointer, Alexander, and Zucker-man, 1995, p. 4).

In the future, governance of the health system (whether it involves multiple boards or not) must support the system's goals, and, if multiple boards are maintained, each must ensure that its operating unit contributes to the system's future success. Further-more, all boards within the system will need to monitor different measures to assess performance—of the system overall, of the oper-ating unit, and of the senior management team. For example, tra-ditional accounting and financial controls should be de-emphasized in favor of a focus on more balanced "performance scorecards," using measures of customer satisfaction, market demand, and com-munity health status.

The complex and duplicative board structures that evolved in health care institutions resulted from attempts to solicit adequate representation from key community leaders—although, within these structures, community representation largely meant input and guidance primarily from the *business* community. Rarely was there more than token representation from physicians, public health, and/or other health-related executives on a system board. In the future, the governing structures of more advanced health care systems will reflect their organizations' commitment to community health with a diversified board whose members understand the delivery of services at different points along the care continuum, not solely the acute care portion.

From a manager's perspective the whole world seems to be turning upside down. Before, successful managers would strive to build their organization's market image and reputation to increase inpatient volumes and demand for high-tech (and high-cost) outpatient services. They focused their efforts on recruiting the best and the brightest super-specialists and purchasing the technology needed to support their practices.

Today the rules of the game have radically changed. Patients are discouraged from receiving care as inpatients unless absolutely medically necessary. Moreover, many of the high-tech services may turn out to be much too costly for the system to own and should instead be divested and contracted for in the future. Furthermore, many managers who have been successful in the past do not understand how they can succeed in this new environment. They may understand in theory where their new emphasis should be, but many simply do not know how to run some of the growing segments of the new health care delivery system's business—including home care, subacute care, and primary care.

Unfortunately, without informed and enlightened leadership, the management team of the past may unintentionally restrict the growth of these new critical activities by allocating too many resources to inpatient services rather than to an expanded continuum of care, especially primary care. This inclination is particularly true of the system "cash cow," which is "usually the flagship of the system and, as such, has often been granted the most autonomy to pursue its own interests" (Shortell, Gillies, and others, 1993, p. 453). What will be imperative for each management team (and governing body) to understand is that "today's 'cash cows' may well become tomorrow's 'dogs,' and continued investment in them to the exclusion of newly emerging priorities could bring down the entire system" (Shortell, Gillies, and others, 1993, p. 453).

Finally, to facilitate the transition, new or evolving systems must clearly *define* the new roles and responsibilities of board members and managers, including physicians. Part of the difficulty in accomplishing change today is that key organizational leaders do not precisely understand how they will fit into the system or where they should direct their attention. It has been said that people pay attention to those activities for which they are rewarded. To encourage new behaviors in the system's key leadership, in particular its management, the reward structure must change. If managers are told to be creative and to take risks, for example, they should no longer remain subject to outmoded performance evaluation systems or inappropriate financial hurdles. One system in the study, for example, significantly altered its incentive compensation program to better reflect its new system goals. In this new program, the operating unit CEOs' bonuses are based on the following: results of their hospitals' cost-reduction initiative (25 percent); results of the system's cost-reduction initiative (25 percent); overall evaluation of how well the CEO has performed with respect to the system's specified list of Core Performance Criteria—supporting the mission, improving quality, providing appropriate incentives to others, and achieving integration (50 percent). In sum, board members and managers should be encouraged to support new business practices with incentives that hold them accountable for their actions through a meaningful relationship between risk and reward.

Inability to Understand and Internalize the New Health Care Environment

Many health care leaders can describe what an organized delivery system is, or should be. However, they tend to stumble when they are expected to "walk the talk." For a system to succeed, capital decisions must be based on a system's ability to develop an integrated continuum of care with primary care at its center. The majority of capital funds must be allocated to primary care rather than to acute care. Further, operating-unit managers must be convinced that building a system around primary health care is viable. They should harbor no confusion about the emphasis on primary care spending.

Managers must also understand that physician integration and primary care physician recruitment are not strategies to feed hospital inpatient business but are key components for negotiating managed care contracts (including capitated contracts that generate system revenue up front). Insightful physician leaders combined with enhanced information systems can make an important difference.

Finally, one cannot overstate the importance of managing the *pace* of the change. Like Wayne Gretzsky, organizations must assess their unique situations and "skate to where the puck will be." However, not overshooting the target—or, in this case, the market—is equally important. Moving an organization too far too fast can be just as disabling as not moving it at all. Consequently, as an organization considers various governance and management models, it should assess in what form and at what speed the market will change, and pursue the new structure with a level of intensity in keeping with that organization's readiness for change.

The most difficult part of this challenge is to accurately assess the market to ensure that the organization will be in the right place at the right time. As noted in Chapter Two, a market moves at different paces depending on its stage of evolution. Clearly, the slowest part of the transformation is early on, as a market is moving from Stage 1 to Stage 2. However, beware of the transition from Stage 2 to Stage 3, for it is likely to occur at breathtaking speed.

The market could change literally overnight as a result of some watershed event. Thus the trick is to move ahead of the market so that the organization is prepared for change, but not so far ahead that it loses its competitive advantage to others who are better meeting current market needs.

Shortage of Talent with the "Right" Skills

Organizations often have difficulty implementing their integration plans not because the plan stems from an incorrect strategy but because managers do not understand the strategy, disagree with it, lack sufficient incentives to motivate action, or lack sufficient skills to implement it. As with so many of these critical hurdles, the skills needed to succeed in the past are not the same skills needed to succeed in the future. Many administrators who grew up in hospitals are uncertain about their new roles and do not fully comprehend the relationship between hospitals, physician partners, other continuum services, payers, managed care products, and communities. If an integrated system is to work, managers must thoroughly understand these relationships. Otherwise they may feel like targets of change rather than agents of change, and may fear (potentially with some reason) that their power and influence are being reduced.

Once the optimal governance and management models have been selected, individuals will dictate how well the infrastructure works. Unfortunately, many of the key system board members and executives have never had to think "system" as opposed to "operating unit," and consequently they may not be as skilled in the new world as they were in the old. Many leaders do not even know what other system operating units *do* or how they contribute to the overall system strategy, which means these leaders will have particular difficulty integrating the units.

Furthermore, as we have noted previously, an essential source of key leadership talent is the organization's physicians. Unfortunately, like managers, few physicians have the right skills to allow them to succeed in leadership roles—including "people" skills, analytical ability, business acumen, "big picture" vision—while also commanding respect among other physicians and staff. Physicians with an appropriate blend of these capabilities are in high demand and difficult to recruit. Consequently, as noted in Chapter Five, organizations must carefully select and groom potential physician leaders so that a pool of candidates will be available to the organization over the long term.

Fear of Losing Control

Historically, boards, managers, and physicians have each retained a reasonable degree of autonomy and control. Today, as the discussion turns to integration and collaboration, health care leaders are not sure what will happen if they give up control. Although distributing control among a variety of leaders and functions can be difficult, studies show that organizations willing to do so seem to function better in changing environments.

The present research shows that both "group" and "developmental" cultures can foster an environment that supports integration. Specifically, a "group" culture—characterized by an emphasis on flexibility and trust, a participatory leadership style, and sensitivity to many viewpoints during decision making—supports integration. Similarly, a "developmental" culture—identified by an emphasis on flexibility, an entrepreneurial and risk-taking leadership style, and empowerment at all levels to facilitate quick decision making—also supports integration. Furthermore, empowerment alone promotes an organization's *transactive memory*, defined as employee and member knowledge of what each other knows (Wegner, 1986). The greater an organization's transactive memory, the greater its ability to diffuse learning throughout the organization and to adapt to a rapidly changing environment (Argote, 1993).

The only way an organization will ever be able to respond quickly to a rapidly changing environment is to loosen the control belt. Indeed, if one looks at the winners of the Malcolm Baldrige Award (which recognizes select organizations nationwide for their success), a hallmark of the leaders of these organizations is their willingness to empower both personnel and partners to best serve their customers. Similarly, a recent case study of ten systems notes that "almost without exception, in the process of becoming a more integrated system, hospital administrators and boards have relinquished a significant share of their authority" (Coddington, Moore, and Fischer, 1994, p. 117).

Fear of Failure

Another key challenge leaders must address is to alleviate the natural fear of failure that boards, managers, and key physicians will inevitably face as the integration process evolves. Over the years, many organizations have enjoyed long traditions of success as a result of their ability to develop and perfect certain characteristics and behaviors. However, when the environment changes, different factors will determine organizations' relative competitive positions. Past success is no longer a valid predictor of future success.

Thus, painful though it may be, organizations must replace the familiar and the comfortable with the unproved. How they cope will vary. One study system leadership team used the following analogy to describe its view of the future, an analogy that also explains their very real fear of failure and the challenges they face in coming to terms with it.

> Imagine that over the years you have become a very successful health care manager. You have continually sped along the road with a vehicle that has been more than adequate to move you forward. Now, suddenly the road stops at a cliff, overlooking a canyon. Others who have reached the cliff before you have begun building a ramp—à la Evil Knevil—to allow you to jump across. However, misty weather obscures the canyon's depth and, more important, its width. Moreover, you cannot see the terrain on the opposite side. Is it smooth, or does

it slope gently downward? Or is it strewn with rocks, or even boulders? The vehicle you have relied on over the years is old and not that powerful. It is, in fact, a 1965 school bus. How confident would you be in racing up the ramp to jump over the canyon?

Managers are being asked to "rev up their engines" and go for it. The experts say that success is theoretically possible. However, no one (not the driver, not the builder of the ramp, not even the cheerleader) really knows whether or not the bus will make it. In a world of tremendous change, taking a giant leap of faith based only on a "trust us" rationale results in an exceedingly justifiable fear of failure. Organizations must both acknowledge that fear and seek to root it out. How successful they are at doing so will affect the organization's long-term success.

Key Success Factors

In the future, providing high-quality health services at competitive costs will be critical. However, organizations will not be capable of achieving this goal "with outmoded organizational systems and processes" (Griffith, 1995, p. 12). Analyses of study participants suggest that the following actions can help an organization build the structures it needs to help break down internal barriers and ensure success: streamline the governance process, redefine management roles, develop strong physician leaders, and implement broader performance accountability criteria.

Streamline the Governance Process

Some suggest that "because of the unique position of boards, governance is potentially the ultimate integrator" (Pointer, Alexander, and Zuckerman, 1995, p. 3). Indeed, the board level is the only place within the system where every piece finally comes together. However, in a fast-paced world, organizations no longer have the luxury of time to evaluate, debate, analyze again, build consensus, and then decide which strategic move makes the most sense. Further, as organizations become more integrated, multiple board structures appear to be unnecessary to the process of governing a single organization striving to accomplish a common goal. Especially where operating units serve a common marketplace, maintaining a segregated, dispersed system of governing may be counterproductive.

Organizations that serve several distinct regions also continue to streamline their governance processes, but they do so by region. In essence, they create a "wide area network (WAN)" at the system level that links together a series of "local area networks (LANs)" within each region. Each market is governed by a streamlined process that has either collapsed all boards into a single, regional corporate board, or dramatically transferred "significant" governing powers to the regional board while delegating specific quality-of-care issues to advisory boards at the individual operating units. During the course of the study, such governing bodies were instituted by at least half of the study systems. Other systems around the country have followed suit. For example, El Camino Health System in Mountain View, California, has concentrated critical system decision making in a shared governance model, featuring a ten-member executive council that includes five physicians (*Medical Care Strategy Report*, 1994).

Redefine Management Roles

Management practices and skills of the past are not necessarily the best skills for the future. In fact, as described in the case study of Sharp HealthCare to follow, replacing the traditional, business-trained health care executive with a manager who is well versed in the system's clinical delivery may make more sense given the manager's key responsibilities in a managed marketplace. Sharp, for example, replaced the CEO of its flagship hospital with a two-person team—a nurse executive and a physician executive. These professionals' strong clinical experience made them highly qualified to determine how best to reengineer the institution's delivery of health care services. Furthermore, they garnered tremendous support from employees and physicians, who felt that "two of their own" were steering the ship.

As with governance, management must be streamlined so that the decision-making process is quick and its organizational structure is nimble enough to rapidly respond to various market dynamics. Most of the study participants experienced numerous management reorganizations during the four years of the study. These changes typically involved combining the management of functions and services *across* the delivery system—essentially breaking down historical barriers and "smokestacks." Often a single individual was appointed as regional manager responsible for the entire continuum of care within a defined geographic area. Hospital CEO positions were eliminated and individuals reassigned to oversee systemwide or regional responsibilities. These efforts generally included integrating all types of care (inpatient and outpatient acute care, primary care, rehabilitative care, and so on) and support functions (human resources, information management, total quality management, and managed care) in a coordinated fashion at the system level. Systems outside our study have taken similar action. Kaiser Permanente of Northern California, for example, has created eight subregions designated as "accountable business units" (Integrated Health Care Report, 1994). These business units are overseen by eight service-area managers responsible for all hospitals and clinics within a given area. As a result of this process, Kaiser has replaced fifteen hospital CEOs.

Finally, systems must also restructure the reward system to provide incentives for important activities and penalties for those that are counterproductive. Many of the study participants' senior managers are rewarded based on overall *system* performance (such as cost reductions, financial results, patient satisfaction, enrollment growth, and system market share), and no longer on the bottom-line performance of their operating unit alone (this latter incentive fosters counterproductive competition among system units). ODSs need their managers to focus on the competition *outside* the system—not within it.

Develop Strong Physician Leaders

As documented in the study and reiterated throughout this book, systems require a nucleus of physician leadership—at the board level, within the senior management team, and within affiliated physician group practices. Systems must identify those physician champions who can lead the charge, provide them with the necessary authority and support to succeed, and adequately reward them for their contributions. (See Chapter Five for additional discussion of this topic.)

Implement Broader Performance Accountability Criteria

As systems become more responsible for the health of enrolled lives and ultimately share in responsibility for the health of the community, they will need to develop broader performance accountability criteria. These criteria should include access, cost, quality, and outcome measures that address the needs of multiple external stakeholder groups, including patients, employers, payers, community groups, regulators, and accreditation bodies, among others. At the same time, systems must develop measures that are useful for internal stakeholders, including physicians, nurses, other health professionals, executives, and board members. Such measures become the raw material for use in report cards and, perhaps more important, the input for interactive control systems (Simons, 1995) that enable organized delivery systems to take real-time corrective action and initiate continuous improvement efforts. Some have referred to these measures as developing *instrument panels* that enable organized delivery systems to manage wisely, much as the cockpit crew on an airplane needs instrument panels to fly safely (Nelson and others, 1995). The approach is similar to the "balanced scorecard" approach adopted by a number of corporations in other fields

(Kaplan and Norton, 1992, 1993). Examples include measures of customer service and satisfaction, quality and outcome of clinical processes, cost and financial performance, growth, and degree of system integration. The list that follows provides some balanced scorecard examples used by the Henry Ford Health System.

Henry Ford Balanced Scorecard Performance Measures

1. External customer satisfaction
   Percent of patients dissatisfied or very
      dissatisfied
   Percent of voluntary disenrollment
   Access indicators
   Physician satisfaction survey
   Business attitude evaluation
2. Clinical process—outcomes
   Accreditation and regulatory approvals
   Health status (SF-36)
   Number of claims and litigations
   Patient falls
   Nosocomial infection rates
   HCFA-derived disease-specific mortality rates
3. Financial performance
   Net operating income
   Cost/enrollee or cost/case (case mix adjusted)
   Patient days/1,000 members
   DRG margin
   Bond rating
4. Philanthropy
   Total donations received (including commitments)
   Net philanthropic collections (net of expenses)
   Philanthropic expense ratio
5. Community dividend
   Uncompensated care
   Contribution in voluntary efforts including such

activities as community education (staff hours,
$ value)

6. Growth
   Equivalent population served
   Market share

7. Business strategic advantage
   Cost leadership
   Distribution system
   Product offerings
   Process improvement teams—accomplishments

8. Innovation
   Percentage revenue from new products
   Percentage revenue from new markets

9. Internal customer satisfaction
   Employee satisfaction surveys
   Labor turnover
   Diversity goals

10. Academic (education and research)
    NIH grants received
    Total external funding
    Resident match results
    Student satisfaction with educational programs
    [Henry Ford Health System, 1995]

The following is an example from July 1994 of the "instrument panel" measures used by the northern region of the Dartmouth Hitchcock Health System.

HIGHLIGHTS Measures of Performance (MSP) Northern Region—July 1994

- *Instrument Panel:*   All customer-based measures remain in statistical control. For the 12 months of FY 1994 the means for these measures range from 61 percent maximum achievable for Community Image, 65 percent for Employee Satisfaction,

75 percent for Patient Satisfaction, and 87 percent for Access.

- *Access:* All respondents scheduling their appointments by telephone rate the ease of this as very good or excellent. More than 7 in 10 respondents were very satisfied with the wait associated with scheduling their appointment and the wait in the exam room.

- *Patient Satisfaction:* About 4 in 10 patients rated overall clinical quality a perfect 10. Bragging edged out complaining by a margin of about 3 to 1.

- *Functional Health Status:* About 3 in 10 respondents rated their overall health as excellent. Between 30 percent and 50 percent of patients reported either some limitations due to physical or emotional problems or some interference with daily work or social activities.

- *Community Image:* Respondents heard more complaints than brags over the past 3 months. This 2 to 1 margin helped to push the composite score below the average percent maximum achievable for the previous 12 months.

- *Employee Satisfaction:* Complaints exceeded brags for nonphysician employees, while the opposite was true for physician responders. This, coupled with slightly lower rating of overall work place quality by physicians, helped in moving the composite score for this month below the average of the prior 12.

- *Management Process:* For both physicians and non-physician groups their immediate supervisors' willingness to let them try new methods was a strength. About 10 percent of nonphysicians rated leadership communication of a clear mission as excellent; none of the physician respondents rated it as excellent.

- *Referring Physician Satisfaction:* The operational definition of this measure has been expanded. Brags outstripped complaints and the rating of the overall referral process ranged from 4 to 10. Six in 10 referring physicians rated access for their patients as excellent. About 4 in 10 rated communication as excellent.

- *Research:* This measure is being reported for the first time this month. Between 15 percent and 20 percent of physician respondents rated administration's support and value of research and their time to do research as very good. Individual physician rating of their own research productivity ranged from 1 to 8, with 10 being the best. The average number of publications identified in print was about 13.

- *Information Systems:* This measure is being reported for the first time this month. Employee ratings of the information systems ranged from 1 to 9 with over 60 percent being 7 or higher.

Operational Definitions including the newly identified measures will be available on the DHMC [Dartmouth-Hitchcock Medical Center] file server in the Measures of System Performance Folder during the month of September.

A copy of the current MSP report will also be available on the DHMC file server in the Measures of System Performance Folder during the month of September.

Description of Measures

- *Access:* Patient satisfaction with access to care from the clinic.

- *Patient Satisfaction:* Patient ratings of quality of care recently received from the clinic.

- *Functional Health Status:* Patient-based data on health status postcare.

- *Community Image:* Community resident view of the goodness of the clinic as a place to receive care.

- *Employee Satisfaction:* Employee ratings of the quality of the clinic as a place to work.

- *Management Process:* Employee ratings of leaders and cooperation.

- *Referring Physician Satisfaction:* Physician ratings of the goodness of DHMC as a place to refer their patients.

- *Volume of Services:* Clinic Outpatient Visits (the sum of Medical and Surgical visits in all Lebanon outpatient locations), Outreach Visits (the sum of visits to all outreach locations), and Admissions (the sum of hospital inpatient, inpatient psychiatric, and newborn admissions).

- *Profitability:* Quarterly and year-to-date net operating income.

- *Research:* Physician rating of support, value, and research productivity.

- *Information Systems:* Employee rating of the information systems. [Nelson and others, 1995, p. 161.]

Figure 7.1 shows some of Mercy Health System's planned measures, which are directly linked to their strategic objectives and goals.

The strength of these performance measurement systems lies in their ability to provide incentives to caregivers, executives, and board members to monitor elements that truly make a difference to the organization's competitive position, while also providing key information useful to external bodies.

Figure 11.1. Mercy Health Services: The Strategic Context of Performance Measures.

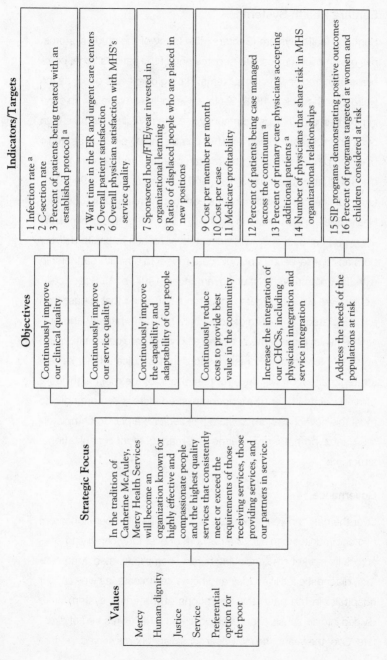

Values

Mercy
Human dignity
Justice
Service
Preferential
option for
the poor

Strategic Focus

In the tradition of
Catherine McAuley,
Mercy Health Services
will become an
organization known for
highly effective and
compassionate people
and the highest quality
services that consistently
meet or exceed the
requirements of those
receiving services, those
providing services, and
our partners in service.

Objectives

Continuously improve
our clinical quality

Continuously improve
our service quality

Continuously improve
the capability and
adaptability of our people

Continuously reduce
costs to provide best
value in the community

Increase the integration of
our CHCSs, including
physician integration and
service integration

Address the needs of the
populations at risk

Indicators/Targets

1 Infection rate [a]
2 C-section rate
3 Percent of patients being treated with an
established protocol [a]

4 Wait time in the ER and urgent care centers
5 Overall patient satisfaction
6 Overall physician satisfaction with MHS's
service quality

7 Sponsored hour/FTE/year invested in
organizational learning
8 Ratio of displaced people who are placed in
new positions

9 Cost per member per month
10 Cost per case
11 Medicare profitability

12 Percent of patients being case managed
across the continuum [a]
13 Percent of primary care physicians accepting
additional patients [a]
14 Number of physicians that share risk in MHS
organizational relationships

15 SIP programs demonstrating positive outcomes
16 Percent of programs targeted at women and
children considered at risk

[a]These are important stretch indicators for the future; as of today, definitional issues are unresolved, therefore, future modifications could be significant.

Source: Reprinted with permission of Mercy Health Services, 1995, p. 6.

Sentara Health System

Sentara Health System (Sentara), like many of the study systems, has grown over the years to become one of the nation's large, comprehensive, regional health systems. Having opened its doors as the Retreat for the Sick in 1888, Sentara has continued to focus on serving the Hampton Roads community in eastern Virginia for more than one hundred years. However, after completing a year-long strategic planning process involving more than one hundred Sentara physicians, voluntary board members, and managers, in mid-1994 Sentara redefined how it will serve its community in the future. Sentara Health System will transform itself into a truly integrated health delivery system and as such will redirect its approach to health delivery from an "illness-based episodic care model to a health partnership with the community" ("New Governance," 1994, p. 1). Specifically, Sentara will strive to create a new model of caring that is based on an "integrated continuum of education, self-care, primary and preventive health management, as well as chronic care coordination and episodic intervention." Sentara leadership has indicated that its new strategic direction will likely represent one of the most significant turning points in Sentara's accomplished history. Accordingly, to meet this new challenge, Sentara has set forth a plan to completely reorganize both its governance and management organizational structures.

Governance

Over the past ten years, Sentara has diversified its operations from two community hospitals to a network of over forty caregiving sites across its market area, including nursing homes, assisted-living centers, diagnostic facilities, day and home health care, as well as four hospitals. In the past, the operations of the entire system were divided into six subsidiaries, each governed by its own board of directors. Over the years, the individual subsidiary boards served Sentara well by providing its various divisions with the necessary level of attention and focus to guide these newly formed and growing businesses through the early stages of their development. When Sentara leadership adopted its new vision, however, it realized the multidivisional structure that had served it well in the past would no longer be appropriate. The strategic planning process showed the need for a singular entity to guide (and govern) the strategic direction of all components of the system. Without such a common structure, Sentara could potentially have separate governing bodies moving the system in conflicting directions. Consequently, the Sentara Health System board voted in July 1994 to consolidate all six of its subsidiary boards into one expanded community board of directors.

To ease the transition, Sentara leadership decided to ask each subsidiary board member to continue to serve Sentara in some manner after the restructuring—either on the expanded Sentara Health System board, as a trustee, or as a director emeritus. The Sentara board of directors has been charged with overseeing the total operation and management of the Sentara Health System. It is composed of fifteen members (eleven volunteer community representatives, three physicians, and the CEO), all of whom also serve as trustees of the corporation. All the traditional governing responsibilities—setting the future direction of the corporation, monitoring its financial performance, and assessing its stewardship of assets for the communities' benefit fall to these fifteen board members.

The trustees of the corporation provide vital linkages to the communities Sentara serves by encouraging a better understanding of Sentara's mission in the community. It is also the trustees' annual responsibility to elect the directors of the corporation. There are approximately thirty trustees of Sentara (with the fifteen directors accounting for nearly half of these trustees).

Further, as part of the governance reorganizational effort, the Sentara board of directors also created a new directors emeritus group, composed of approximately fifty volunteer community leaders who "provide valuable insight and wisdom to Sentara as well as to the community by serving as liaisons between Sentara and the region it serves" ("New Governance," 1994, p. 1). As described by E. George Middleton Jr., Sentara's chairman of the board of directors, Sentara is looking to this key group of community leaders as one way to provide the inspiration needed to impact the health of the community and respond to needs for quality and cost-efficient care. Finally, as with most study participants, Sentara has also concluded that the integration of physicians into the governance of its system will be critical to the success of the new organization.

Management

Sentara completely reorganized its management structure as part of the strategic planning process. (Figure 7.2 shows Sentara's recent organizational chart.) Like its initial board structure, Sentara's management structure had been organized along functional lines—with one division devoted to alternative delivery systems (which included Sentara's Health Plan) and the other five divisions devoted to its "delivery system," which included its hospitals, life care facilities (nursing homes and assisted-living facilities), and health enterprises. Like many systems around the country, physicians in the Sentara system were always critically important, but they did not play a significant formal role in the management of the system. Sentara recognized that true physician integration would be critical to its future success and has responded by substantially increasing the formal role of physicians throughout the system.

In place of that more traditional system, Sentara formed a new executive council to serve its whole organization. The council reports to Sentara's CEO and serves as the CEO's key strategy advisory team. The group, as a whole, has no direct line responsibilities; however, some of the management council members do have line responsibility for a number of Sentara businesses. The primary role of the executive council is to ensure the long-term development and viability of Sentara as a health management company. To do this the council has been charged with the following:

Figure 7.2. Management Structure of Sentara Health System.

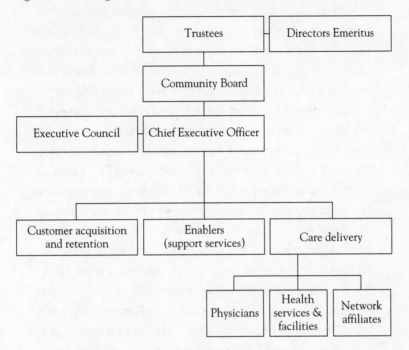

- Fulfilling the organization's mission
- Leading as agents of change
- Promoting excellence in system operations and health care delivery
- Creating a competitive advantage
- Growing and retaining the business
- Maintaining the fiscal strength of the system
- Planning for the future

Since the group does not have the line responsibility to accomplish many of these charges, members instead serve as catalysts for the desired changes, monitor progress in these areas, and determine if the system needs to modify its strategic direction.

To support Sentara's commitment to become more of a physician-driven organization, the newly formed executive council is composed of an equal number of executives and physicians—four of each. The CEO selected the four management representatives who sit on the council while the physician representatives were chosen following an intensive application and interview process. Of the four physician members selected, two are primary care practitioners and two are specialists, and all continue to maintain active medical practices. Each physician council member devotes approximately thirty-two hours a month to council duties. Sentara envisions that in the future the executive council physician members will be committed full-time to council activities, either through a contractual or employment relationship. Furthermore, as the new structure evolves, the physician members will likely be accountable for significant operating responsibilities as are their management counterparts. Toward that end, one of the council physician members has been appointed vice president and chief medical officer; as such, he will devote more than 70 percent of his time to such management responsibilities as medical management, outcomes management, and clinical integration, and will serve as CEO of Sentara's Medical Group.

In addition to creating the eight-member executive council, Sentara continues to streamline and reorganize the balance of its management structure. One such change includes the reduction of the number of levels of personnel (particularly management personnel) within the Sentara system. Sentara has recently set as its target to have no more than four to five levels of personnel throughout the entire system, including the CEO, system vice presidents, functional managers or process leaders, and front line personnel (including working supervisors). The significant reduction of system costs is clearly one of the primary motivating factors of this reorganizational effort. Indeed, Sentara believes that this streamlining process, coupled with the implementation of more efficient technologies and processes, will enable it to reduce costs between $95 and $100 million over the next three to five years.

To better enable the system to function as a truly integrated company—rather than as a combination of its many parts—Sentara has split its entire organization into two core business processes: (1) customer acquisition and retention and (2) care delivery. The Customer Acquisition and Retention division includes such functional areas as marketing and sales, product and network design, and claims and servicing. The Care Delivery division includes the following activities and services:

- Physicians—aligned within one of three different models: Sentara Medical Group (SMG), the independent physician association (IPA), or as medical staff with privileges

- Health services and facilities—hospitals, urgent care facilities, nursing homes, and home health

- Network affiliates (such as non-owned but related Sentara hospitals, pharmacies, physicians, and medical schools)

Furthermore, like many companies in other industries, Sentara has adopted a team approach to manage each division. Rather than having a single individual overseeing the complex and diverse operations included within each division, Sentara has assigned several vice presidents to run each of these two divisions.

To support these two core business processes, Sentara identified "Enabler Teams" that encompass most traditional support services that both divisions need in order to function smoothly—including finance, human resources, information systems, facilities support, and related areas. Leaders of each of these areas are responsible for their function throughout the system (regardless of the specific site or location). For example, the vice president of human resources is in charge of all human resources personnel, issues, and functions systemwide. Furthermore, all human resources personnel throughout the system will be assigned to one of five human resources teams—each specializing in a particular area but serving the entire system. The planned human resources teams cover organizational entry, compensation and benefits, training and development, compliance and regulations, and operational support (generalists who serve each Sentara operating unit). Moreover, to ensure that the Enabler Teams adequately and appropriately serve the various operating units and processes, Sentara will use service agreements to outline the specific service each operating unit needs and expects from each member of the Enabler Teams. This agreement will be revised periodically to ensure that it outlines current system needs and is used as one way to regularly evaluate the performance of the Enabler Team members.

In addition to streamlining the number of levels and divisions within its system, Sentara has also put in place new initiatives that allow it to begin to better coordinate functions across the system. Over the next few years Sentara will consolidate all clinical support functions (such as pharmacy, laboratory, and radiology) at the system level. For example, Sentara plans to aggregate all pharmacy activities, with only "interim and STAT dose" pharmacies located on site in each operating unit. The same strategy is planned for the laboratory: a single reference laboratory will serve all Sentara operating units, with only "rapid response" laboratory capabilities located at each operating unit (including Norfolk General, Sentara's flagship tertiary hospital).

Consolidation also applies to professional service contracts. Sentara envisions that it will contract with only one physician group for each of its hospital-based professional services (including pathology, emergency medicine, anesthesiology, and radiology). In other words, only one group of pathologists would be responsible for covering (or subcontracting with others to cover) all pathology service needs throughout the Sentara system (including each Sentara hospital and outpatient surgical site).

Thus, Sentara is currently implementing a radically new way of organizing to facilitate the achievement of its integration goals. Each new initiative reflects Sentara's commitment to creating a new organization that will operate as a single entity—a goal that is both supported and encouraged by the findings in our study. As with many new changes, some initiatives will likely be more effective than others. Consequently, Sentara's current integration approach will certainly undergo many iterations as it strives to provide more cost-effective care to its communities.

Sharp HealthCare

Over the course of the study, Sharp HealthCare (Sharp) embarked on one of the most dramatic organizational changes of any of the study participants. At the study's inception, Sharp was structured similarly to many multihospital health care organizations, using the holding-company model. It had a parent company—the San Diego Hospital Association—which had both a governing board and a number of corporate managers. Reporting to that parent company board were the boards of directors of each of Sharp's individual operating units— its five hospitals, two physician groups, two senior health corporations, and its foundation. Furthermore, each operating unit had its own management team, personnel, services, and functions. There was relatively little integration across the system when the study began in 1990.

Governance

Sharp's general structure of governance has not radically changed over the past several years. It has actively reemphasized the critical importance of maintaining a special connection with each community its operating units serve, and it has chosen a community-based board as the best way to maintain those relationships. However, to enhance its ability to respond nimbly to the ever-changing San Diego marketplace, Sharp has altered the roles its various boards play. It has concentrated most of the traditional governance powers in the parent board, which sets the systemwide strategic direction, determines system policies, and maintains charge of system fiduciary responsibilities.

The operating-unit boards, in contrast, ensure that each operating unit supports the overall policies and strategic direction set by the parent board. These boards address such specific local issues as monitoring the quality of care provided at the local operating unit, overseeing the mission effectiveness of its operating unit, and advising the parent board as to how initiatives may be perceived by the local community and keeping the parent board in touch with that community.

Furthermore, Sharp maintains local ties by including on the parent board representatives from each of the communities its operating units serve. Also, to facilitate integration with its key constituent—the physician—both the parent board and the operating-unit boards comprise a large number of active physicians.

Changes in Sharp's governance structure have been minimal. Transitioning traditionally reserved powers from the operating units to the parent board, thereby essentially creating advisory boards at the local level, occurred slowly and with much education. When the changes were finally implemented at Sharp, they were perceived positively.

Sharp has no plans to radically change its governance structure. However, over time the organization will continue to evaluate the need for separate operating-unit advisory boards.

Management

To create a more nimble organization, Sharp streamlined the traditional hierarchical, smokestack management structure of its hospitals. From the front line employee to the CEO, Sharp has just six levels of personnel:

- Front-line individuals—the people delivering the care or service to the patient or other Sharp employees (for example, front-line human resources personnel dedicated to addressing or triaging questions and/or problems at each operating unit).
- Operations coordinators—working supervisors who are also assigned to specific operating units and spend at least 20 percent of their time delivering the service they are supervising.

- Directors—the first tier of management within the Sharp system. They are responsible for all activities within their departments *across* the institutional division of the system, including preparing and monitoring departmental budgets.

- Vice presidents and/or entity leaders (actual title may vary among operating units)—vice presidents are responsible for multiple functions, all of which cut across the five hospital operating units; entity leaders are responsible for the activities within a single hospital operating unit.

- Senior vice presidents—responsible for nonclinical support functions across the system or for all operations within a single division of the system.

- Chief executive officer—responsible for all activities within the system.

Through this streamlined approach, Sharp has been able to eliminate half (or 120) of its hospital management positions.

More specifically, Sharp has aggregated all nonclinical support functions at the system level, including finance, human resources, planning, marketing and public relations, business transactions, fundraising, quality and mission, information systems, and facility development. All personnel within these functional areas report solely to the lead individual for that area. Furthermore, each operating unit has a number of generalists representing nonclinical support functions who answer and/or triage questions and problems to the appropriate system functional specialists. In addition, Sharp has consolidated all its operations into two system divisions—institutional (hospital) or ambulatory (including physician activities and practices)—each of which is led by a single senior executive. (Figure 7.3 shows Sharp's recent organizational chart.)

Management within the institutional operations division acknowledged that in the near future, Sharp probably would not need more than eight hundred acute care beds systemwide. Therefore, rather than duplicate the full complement of managers and/or services

Figure 7.3. Management Structure of Sharp HealthCare.

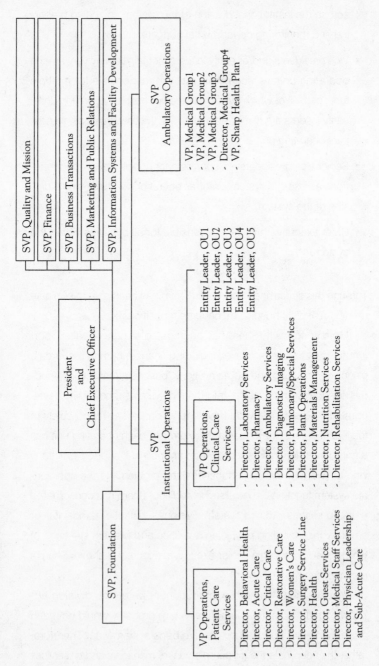

at each of Sharp's five hospitals—which would only represent, on average, approximately 160 beds each—Sharp created a systemwide management team responsible for all 800 beds in the institutional division.

Sharp created a team of two vice presidents to oversee the operations of its five hospitals, ultimately choosing two nurses based on their provider-based understanding of the business and their demonstrated leadership. Each vice president is responsible for approximately ten directors, who manage their particular functions across the entire system. For example, the director of radiology is responsible for all radiology (inpatient and outpatient) at each of the five hospital locations; likewise the director of critical care is responsible for all critical care services throughout the Sharp system. Each director is in turn responsible for all employees within his or her department, no matter which hospital operating unit the employee calls home. Finally, consistent with a streamlined approach to delivering services, Sharp has distributed the operational vice presidents and the functional directors throughout the system rather than move all "management" to the central corporate office. This approach eliminates unnecessary corporate overhead and places key management personnel at all hospital operating units.

Furthermore, to ensure that each hospital's operations continue to run smoothly, as well as to maintain positive community relations, Sharp created a new entity leader position at each hospital operating unit. The entity leader is charged with managing the hospital's board processes and is the primary Sharp management representative with whom the local board relates. This individual is the key liaison between management and that hospital's medical staff, attending medical executive committee and other key medical staff meetings and being available to discuss concerns of the medical staff. Finally, the entity leader is the primary person responsible for facilitating solutions to interdepartmental problems. Although no personnel report to the entity leader, he or she is responsible for ensuring that problems are satisfactorily addressed by the appropriate functional director(s) or operational vice president(s).

Sharp was initially concerned about how the boards, medical staff, and employees would respond to a person with no direct line responsibility. The reaction to date has been quite positive. Some speculate that this positive reaction can be attributed to the entity leader's having a stronger focus on a limited scope of responsibilities. The board members, especially, appreciate having a key manager with more time to devote to their concerns. Likewise medical staff also benefit from greater access to a key system manager.

Finally, Sharp recently instituted a program to address some key activities across the entire system, including its institutional, ambulatory, and corporate divisions. Management realized that in its effort to eliminate the smokestacks among the various operating units, it had created two large smokestacks representing the two operational divisions of the system. To minimize this effect, Sharp identified a number of core processes that it must address systemwide to enhance its competitive position, including customer service, acquisition, and retention; health management; and service line development. Each core process is being addressed by a team of individuals from both operating divisions as well as by some corporate personnel.

One of the initial changes Sharp made was to combine the management teams of two hospitals located near one another. When deciding who would be best qualified to run this combined hospital, senior management first considered what role the hospital played in the system. Through this reflective process management realized that the hospital was simply the inpatient piece of a full continuum of services. In particular, it was an aggregation of a series of nursing units and a place for physicians to deliver their inpatient services. Consequently, Sharp opted to replace the traditional hospital CEO position with a nurse-physician team. This team has recently been absorbed into the systemwide institutional management team.

This innovative and creative approach to redesigning the Sharp management structure was a wake-up call for managers throughout the system. Though many knew of the plans to streamline the management structure and closely reexamine the roles individuals played in the system, most did not fully comprehend the degree of change planned until this seminal event. With this single move, Sharp leadership was able to instantaneously communicate that how Sharp had been structured and managed in the past does not necessarily relate to how it will be organized and managed in the future. Initially combining two hospitals' management teams also allowed Sharp to test the concept of a single management team for all Sharp hospitals and of enhanced dependence on clinical (nurse and/or physician) managers for key senior management roles.

As described above, the ambulatory operations division has not yet been functionally integrated with the institutional division, and the two divisions have duplicative pharmacy, laboratory, surgery services, and personnel. Sharp clearly intends to integrate all functions across the entire system (not just within a single division) over the long term.

Sharp will also continue to focus on creating systems, processes, and standards that will encourage coordination and cooperation among all the functional and clinical pieces of the business—particularly by creating cross-functional and cross-divisional teams devoted to reengineering how Sharp delivers its core processes.

Sisters of Providence–Oregon

Founded in 1856, the Sisters of Providence Health System (Providence) is one of the nation's oldest health systems. Headquartered in Seattle, Washington, Providence has health-related facilities and services (hospitals, physician offices, outpatient centers, long-term care facilities, and health maintenance organizations) throughout Washington, Oregon, California, and Alaska—states that have created and continue to experiment with radically different approaches to health care reform. As health care delivery and management have generally become more responsive to market demands, Providence's leadership recognized that its operating units' strategies, goals, and specific management targets would vary dramatically based on widely dissimilar marketplace conditions and state reform approaches.

Consequently, it chose to create "mini" organized delivery systems within each service area rather than trying to develop an integrated health care delivery system across the entire system.

Providence's operations in Oregon were uniquely well positioned to pilot this regionalization concept. Providence is a significant player in the delivery of health care within Portland and, to a more limited extent, throughout Oregon. Providence has a full complement of health care services along the care continuum in Portland as well as a variety of operating units statewide, and it owns managed care plans in both Washington and Oregon.

Portland itself provides a strong proving ground. Recognized as one of the most efficient health care markets in the country, Portland is also one of the more mature managed care markets. In 1993, Oregon had "the lowest inpatient hospital days-per-thousand of population in the nation—464.9, 44 percent less than the national average" on an age-adjusted basis ("Progressive Portland," 1995, p. 118). Moreover, "on an age-adjusted basis, Oregon . . . ranks 49th in the nation in annual per-capita hospital expenses . . . [and] the Portland/Vancouver/Washington metropolitan area has the highest HMO penetration in the country—63 percent as of January 1994" ("Progressive Portland," 1995, p. 118). Moreover, in February 1994 the state implemented its highly publicized plan for universal coverage, the Oregon Health Plan. Since the plan's inception, the state has been funneling hundreds of thousands of Medicaid recipients into "accountable providers" serving the region. As a result, the Oregon marketplace has emerged as one of the most managed and competitive health care markets in the country.

Each of the market's three major systems—Legacy Health System, Kaiser Permanente's Oregon region, and Sisters of Providence–Oregon—have pursued different strategies to ensure survival and, ultimately, success as Portland's health care provider of choice. In 1994, the Sisters of Providence Health System determined that to respond to the increasing competitive pressures in the Oregon market it had to integrate its Oregon operations. The following sections describe how Providence has organized its units in Portland, Oregon, to operate as a "subsidiary" organized delivery system. (This case study does not address the Sisters of Providence operations outside Oregon.)

Governance

Sisters of Providence organized its Oregon operations around four service areas—Portland, Medford, Seaside, and Newberg—each reflecting the natural physician referral–patient migration pattern around the various operating units. Because Providence's Oregon operations are concentrated primarily within greater metropolitan Portland, Providence–Oregon began its governance-level integration initiatives in that region.

Providence has consolidated the boards of all its operating units—including three hospitals, home services, child care, long-term care, and employed physician practices—into a single community board. The new board overseeing Providence's Portland activities is composed of twenty-one members, seven of whom are physicians. The board is advisory in nature and reports to the policy-setting system board based in Seattle. Medical staff credentialing and quality and safety issues have been fully delegated to the Portland community board by the system board.

Unlike Portland, the other Oregon service areas are each composed of just one or two operating units, such as a hospital and a physician group. Consequently, Providence has not perceived a need to collapse multiple boards within these service areas to create boards comparable to that established in Portland.

In addition, the boards of Providence's two health plans—Vantage (PPO) and Good Health Plan (HMO)—have remained independent from a governance standpoint but have integrated management functions whenever feasible. The health plans serve state residents beyond the service areas in which Providence has providers. Where Providence providers are available, the health plans and the institutions must work cooperatively, but no formal governance relationship exists between the various boards. Thus, from a governance perspective, Providence has established only a "dotted-line" relationship between its health plans and its providers. The health plan boards have been delegated considerable autonomy, with only a few reserved powers held by the system's parent board in Seattle.

Today, Providence–Oregon is evaluating how to better organize the governance of all its operations. Numerous boards throughout the state report directly to the system's parent board; as the state continues to become more managed care oriented and the market more competitive, aligned governance that strategically coordinates all of Providence's Oregon activities (including its managed care efforts) may become increasingly necessary. Attempts continue to be made to better coordinate the health plan and service area boards.

Management

Sisters of Providence–Oregon has also been restructuring its management so that it may function in a more coordinated fashion. (Figure 7.4 shows Providence–Oregon's recent organizational chart). The vice president for operations/Oregon reports directly to the president of the Sisters of Providence Health System. Reporting to the vice president for operations/Oregon are four service area executives who direct operations in each of Providence's four service areas, as well as a group of senior individuals who oversee key local functional and specialty areas including managed care, medical groups, financial services, information services, human resources, planning/government relations, and consulting/auditing.

As with its governance restructuring, Providence–Oregon has primarily focused management reorganization efforts within its Portland operations. The Portland region's first strategic plan, completed in 1990 (Southwick, 1994), showed that operations were both too fragmented and too expensive. It also showed that primary competitors were quickly integrating or consolidating their operations to improve efficiency. As a result, Providence adopted the following goals:

Figure 7.4. Management Structure of Sisters of Providence–Oregon.

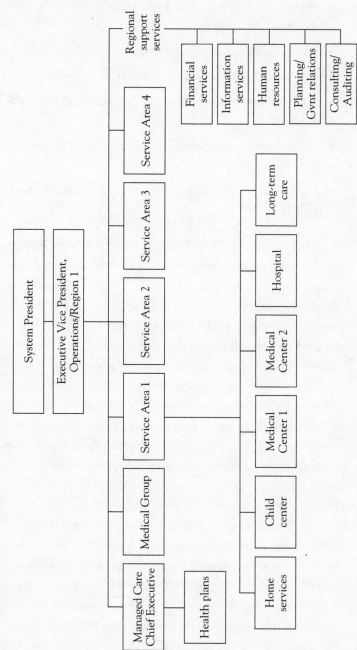

- Provide better coordinated care across delivery sites and providers

- Improve access to primary care providers in the community

- Increase health education and prevention

- Reduce paperwork and facilitate care through an electronic medical record

- Provide patients with better information to help them choose treatment options

- Provide more chronic and long-term services (Southwick, 1994, pp. 2–3)

One of Providence's initial challenges was to change the Portland service area emphasis from one that was "hospital-centric" to a *system* truly focused on its community. To achieve this goal, as described above, Providence installed a single executive who is ultimately responsible for all of the Portland operations, thus eliminating the need for a chief executive over each of its three hospitals; the operating officers of each hospital report to the same regional executive. In addition, traditional department head positions were replaced with service line managers responsible for specific operations at each of the region's operating units—three hospitals, primary care, long-term care, home care, and others. In essence, Providence-Portland created a single management team to manage all Providence operations within Portland and to support the affiliation of smaller service areas throughout Oregon (Southwick, 1994).

This philosophy also applies to the clinical and medical direction at the various Portland campuses. For example, one physician oversees all three emergency rooms, another oversees all three inpatient laboratories, and yet another directs the mental health programs at all three hospitals. Furthermore, Providence-Portland is currently working with a group of Portland-based physicians to develop common clinical pathways and protocols for the operating units. No clinical reconfiguration or consolidation has taken place yet. However, as this regional system evolves, some clinical services will likely be consolidated to a single site.

Providence also organized a variety of shared system support services—such as finance, management information services (MIS), and human resources—to support all service areas throughout Oregon. It aggregated finance, for example, at the state level so that the system could develop economies of scale in accounts receivable management and to assist in statewide managed care contracting. At the operating unit level, financial specialists are available throughout the state to assist personnel on more routine issues.

Management information services are also organized fundamentally at the state level, a structure that enables the MIS department to facilitate the development and implementation of common information systems throughout the state, including the health plans. This approach also enhances the coordination of technology between the Oregon operations and the system overall. To adequately respond to the many issues surrounding information systems technology, technology support personnel are used within each service area.

Human resources have also been aggregated to the state level; however, because issues vary among service areas, some human resources personnel are deployed within each service area to respond to employee questions. Like some of the other study systems, Providence-Oregon will create service agreements to define and then monitor the ongoing service the support teams provide.

Sisters of Providence Health System has made significant strides in achieving its goals, and, in the process, it has come to appreciate its tremendous progress and better understand the level of complexity involved in its work ahead. Integrating a health system is difficult, requiring a great deal of time and generating extreme emotions—"in the end everybody has to change" (Southwick, 1994, p. 7). Like other systems around the country, Providence is forging new ground, knowing that time alone will tell the success of its strategy.

Sutter Health

Sutter Health (Sutter) describes itself as an integrated health care organization (IHO) that serves a diverse set of communities throughout northern California. Sutter provides a full continuum of care across a broad geographic distribution of products and services. Sutter believes that aggregating a comprehensive network of health care services under a common administrative umbrella will "become the principal care delivery structure in the next millennium because of its ability to maintain and strengthen care quality while cutting costs and improving access. As [Sutter] sees it, by managing the diverse parts of the health care delivery system, integrated organizations can more effectively and efficiently manage each patient as their care needs fluctuate during health and illness. That translates into better treatment—a plus for the patient—and fewer dollars spent on expensive, potentially inappropriate, services—a plus in controlling health care costs" ("President's Message," 1992, p. 2).

As Sutter management examined the historical migration patterns of its patients, it saw that the system encompasses several natural boundaries that patients typically did not cross for routine medical care. Consequently, Sutter organized into three regions to accommodate both its size and its broad geographic presence throughout northern California while striving to achieve its vision. Sutter believes its new regional approach will enable it to better serve the unique needs of the communities within each region. Sutter's regions are composed of the operating units (or affiliates, as Sutter refers to them) that have been located within the region historically. The regions—which include aligned physician organizations, hospitals, outpatient facilities, and other services—actually exhibit characteristics of small IHOs.

Governance

A 1987 corporate reorganization created Sutter Health, which serves as the sole corporate member for Sutter's owned facilities. Sutter

Health is governed by a board of directors composed of seven members who are national and regional leaders in business and/or health care. One of the seven board members is also a practicing physician.

Unlike its management structure (described in greater detail below), Sutter has not yet adopted a governance structure that corresponds with its recent regionalization of management. Today, most operating units continue to have dedicated governing bodies that monitor their particular activities. Consequently, to facilitate a culture of systemness at the governance level, Sutter has put in place several different approaches that have proved beneficial. First, Sutter limits its parent-board directors to those who have previously served as directors on one of its affiliate boards. Sutter believes this experience is essential both to orient the parent-board members to critical health care issues and to introduce them to the specifics of the Sutter Health system. Second, all parent-board directors must continue to serve as board members on one of Sutter's affiliates throughout their terms on the parent board. This approach provides the affiliates with an easy means of communicating with the parent board and keeps the parent-board members in touch with the affiliates' local issues. Third, Sutter Health expects its parent-board directors to attend a specified set of affiliate board meetings throughout the year. This structure allows Sutter to maintain an important communication channel to and from affiliates that do not have parent trustees serving on their boards. This arrangement also helps underscore to affiliates their importance to the system.

To facilitate systemness at the governance level, which includes creating a more coordinated approach to the systemwide distribution of resources, Sutter has created planning committees that fit with its regional organization. For each of Sutter's three regions, a Regional Resource Planning Committee (RRPC) has been formed of trustees, physicians, and managers from Sutter facilities within that particular planning region. The RRPC reviews all resource requests to ensure that, at least within the region, resources are used in the most appropriate and effective manner (for example, to enhance

Sutter's competitive position or to realize the best estimated return on investment). This regional approach applies to both the strategic and the capital planning processes. The three RRPCs report to a Systemwide Resource Planning Committee (SRPC), which actually makes the resource allocation decisions for the entire system. The SRPC is composed of representatives from each of the three RRPCs as well as the parent board.

Sutter Health continues to evaluate and fine-tune its governance and management structures. It anticipates that the governance structure may require modification as a result of the study conclusions. One preliminary finding from a related study showed that Sutter's current board structure (which allows each affiliate to maintain its own independent board of directors) costs Sutter approximately $2.5 million annually to staff—in particular, to develop independent financial statements. Therefore, in at least one region where its affiliates serve a common or overlapping market, Sutter anticipates that the boards may be combined in some manner. However, it also acknowledges that combining boards of affiliates that in fact serve unique markets makes little sense—meaning that a number of affiliates would probably not alter their current structure to any great extent.

Management

Sutter has found that as its market has become more "managed," the lines that distinguish the different units have become blurred, making independent management of its various operating units increasingly difficult. Consequently, as briefly mentioned above, Sutter has organized the management of its system around three regions—specifically, the Bay, Central, and Pacific regions. (Figure 7.5 shows Sutter's recent organizational chart.)

Because each region comprises the operating units, which are located within its defined geographic area, each is unique in its service offerings and, perhaps more important, in the issues it must address. For example, Sutter's Central region provides a full continuum of care, including inpatient acute care, outpatient programs,

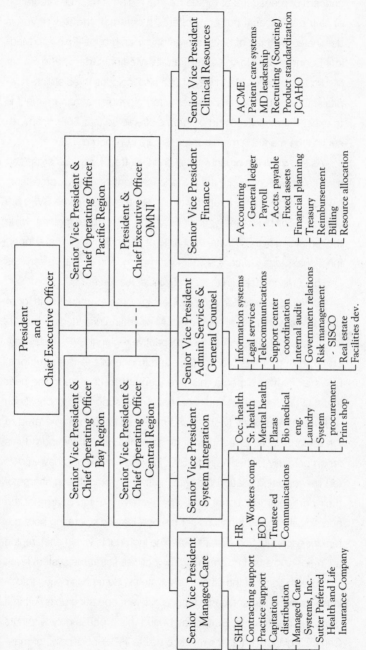

Figure 7.5. Management Structure of Sutter Health.

home health, and physician services. Consequently, the overriding concern of management for the Central region is the true integration of all the services it currently offers. In contrast, the Bay region is dominated by three of Sutter's large physician groups (Palo Alto Medical Foundation, North Coast Faculty Medical Group, and Sutter Medical Foundation North Bay), but it also includes three affiliate hospitals. One of the primary concerns for this region's management is to expand the services and programs offered so that Sutter can present to the market a more complete care continuum.

As shown in the organizational chart, Sutter Health has organized all of its operations under the guidance of eight senior vice presidents (SVPs)—each of whom reports directly to the CEO. Three SVPs are each responsible for the operations of one of the three regions, while the remaining five SVPs are in charge of primarily nonclinical support functions: managed care, system integration, administrative services and general counsel, finance, and clinical resources.

Each regional senior vice president is ultimately responsible for *all* operations within his or her region. All operating unit leaders (including affiliate CEOs) report to their respective regional SVP. (Today several operating units are not included in one of the three regions; however, Sutter expects this arrangement to change in the near future.) Furthermore, all traditional nonclinical support functions (such as human resources, finance, and planning) have been elevated to the regional level. Like the operating unit leaders, these individuals report primarily to their regional SVP. However, many also have a dotted-line reporting relationship with the system executive in charge of their particular functional area. The system SVPs in charge of the nonclinical support functions set the policies and operating parameters for each function systemwide. The individuals within each region are responsible for implementing the policies set at the system level.

As with some of the other study systems, Sutter has begun to collapse its management teams among different operating units within a given region. To date, Sutter has begun this process only within its Central region, which is the most complete IHO. Specifically, for managers of the various functional and operational areas of its two flagship hospitals in downtown Sacramento, Sutter has recently transitioned from two separate management teams to a single management team with functional and operational responsibilities spanning both institutions. This change has allowed Sutter to manage the institutions more efficiently while also transitioning from a traditional system of independent hospitals to an interdependent, coordinated health care system within the Central region. Sutter may consider similar structures within other regions to enhance its system effectiveness and create a more unified approach to serving the region.

Sutter continues to adjust its management and governance structures in the face of rapid and dynamic change in the Northern California health care marketplace. Furthermore, Sutter has stated that its structure will continue to be somewhat fluid in order to rapidly respond and adapt to continually changing market pressures.

Future Challenges

Most organizations today are focusing their efforts on assembling the right pieces. Eventually, however, they will need to determine how to make these pieces work together effectively. The critical choice at that point will be selecting the preferred model of integration—along with the governance and management structures that serve as fundamental building blocks.

Whichever model is pursued, the central goal is to strike a balance among an ODS's three key players—physicians, institutional providers (hospitals, home health agencies, long-term care facilities, ambulatory care settings, and so on), and health plans. In successful systems, these elements maintain equilibrium through aligned or common governance, management, and financial incentives that reward the players for appropriately matching medical resources with the needs of payers and patients (Bartling, 1995). Two approaches commonly employed to achieve this balance are to include leaders from each of these key system components on the senior management team of the system and to create incentives for each leader that encourage cooperation—rather than competition—among the various divisions.

Another key strategic challenge ODSs will face in the future will be to amass the appropriate talent to succeed. In particular, leaders and managers in this new world of health care will require a radically different skill set than that of their predecessors. Some of these "new world" skills include systems thinking, negotiation, conflict management, change management, continuous quality improvement, team building, and network/relationship management. Furthermore, the leader must also be an implementer (not just a visionary).

Implementing systems of care that promote integration across the continuum also requires capital. In the future, the capital for such system development will come less from the operating margins of the system and more from strategic alliances and partnerships with others. Some of those alliances may involve totally new relationships among suppliers—biotech companies, device companies, and pharmaceutical companies—and delivery systems, particularly given that the former have significant sums of capital available relative to the latter.

Systems must also encourage experimentation at all levels. The new "business" of health care must be almost continually reinvented, particularly at those times when one's objectives have been achieved, rapid growth prevails, and one's own organization or one's collaborators and competitors experience unexpected success or failure (Drucker, 1994). ODSs of the future will have neither the luxury to establish fixed rules nor the time to systematically evaluate each move. An organization may establish parameters, but all personnel should have the flexibility, authority, and empowerment to respond quickly to situations as they arise. The organization will benefit from experimenting, learning, and experimenting some more to continuously improve service quality. An ODS's governance and management structures and its physician leadership must promote and support such behavior.

Finally, many systems are beginning to realize that each governance or management model presents a series of trade-offs, and the decisions associated with choosing one can be tremendously difficult and pose serious consequences. What are the short-term political costs of implementing various models? What are the ramifications for the organization if a particular model is not implemented? What is the best timing to implement a change? Must it happen today, or can it wait? Will a given model provide room for future growth and change? Most important, does the management and governance structure support the clinical caregiving process? If not, the net result may be structures whose components are not truly integrated and thus cannot work together.

8

Moving Forward

Policy Issues and Implementation Challenges

Aside from direct public policy intervention (Medicare legislation in 1965 and DRG payment reform in 1983, for example), the primary determinant of the evolution of the U.S. health care system over the past thirty years has been new technology. But looking ahead to the next thirty years, technological forces will be joined by the information explosion, sweeping demographic changes, a restructured work force, increasing social and economic disparities, and a growing demand for value as major shapers of the U.S. health system. The central question is whether these forces will serve to further increase the fragmentation of health care delivery or whether they can somehow be harnessed to reduce fragmentation. New diagnostic, therapeutic, and information technologies have the potential to either fragment or integrate. Demographic diversity and social and economic disparities tend to increase fragmentation. A restructured work force holds potential for further integration. An increased interest in value is likely to result in a greater demand for integration. In this chapter, we discuss the role of organized delivery systems within the context of these forces, whether public policy should encourage the growth of such systems, and how such systems might be held accountable.

Technological Change

The march of biomedical science is relentless. New diagnostic and therapeutic techniques will continue to proliferate, creating enormous pressures on the social and managerial sciences to ensure that the technologies are well utilized and serve the public good. Emphasis will be placed on cost-reducing technologies or at least those that can meet cost-effectiveness and cost/benefit tests (Office of Technology Assessment, 1994). Examples include continued advances in image-guided therapy in which surgeons are able to see into and through patients' bodies; "trackless" surgery in which procedures are performed without touching the body through use of ultrasound waves; the development of surgical robots; genetic engineering, which will usher in an era of "predict and prevent" medicine; gene therapy; and, of course, continued advances in drug therapy ("The Future of Medicine," 1994). Many of these technologies should result in more efficient, less invasive, and quicker positive outcomes for patients. But whether these potential outcomes are achieved depends very much on *how broadly* their implications are viewed. This will depend on the extent to which *information* regarding these new technologies is widely shared among caregivers, settings of care, patients, and the community at large. If these new technologies result in increased concentration of power among a few professional specialties, then the god of fragmentation will be served. But if these new technologies result in a sharing of power among members of the health care team, a greater understanding of the post-intervention care needs of patients, a sensitivity to the ethical choices involved, and, most important, an increase in the empowerment of patients, then the goddess of integration will be served. The issue is not whether technology will continue to provide new advances: the issue is whether technology can be used to integrate rather than divide, whether technology can be managed to serve the public good. The hypothesis is that where communities are served by organized delivery systems with linkages throughout the community, there is a greater likelihood that technological breakthroughs will be integrated into the overall continuum of care than in communities where such systems do not exist.

Information Explosion

We are bombarded by information from the moment we wake up with our clock radio until we watch the evening news before retiring. Information technology joins with scientific technology to rapidly diffuse biomedical innovations throughout the country and, most important, in the minds of all Americans. Rarely a day goes by in which one new diagnostic or therapeutic breakthrough, if not several, are reported by the media. As is the case with biomedical breakthroughs, the information explosion has the potential to either fragment the delivery of health care or result in greater integration of care. The key lies in developing social and managerial architecture that can maintain the emerging technologies in a productive relationship to each other. The information technologies must be treated as servants to the overall vision and strategy of producing coordinated care for patients and health for the community. If coordinated properly, information technology developments will increase the ability of the system to deal with the new biomedical advances by being able to readily evaluate their cost and benefit from a continuum of care and lifetime perspective. New information technologies will also affect how the care itself is provided. Consider the following scenario:

> Picture the new age health care consumer in 2010. In the 1990s an average person would visit a doctor four or five times a year. By 2010 or probably well before that, doctors will be on call via home personal computers, through electronic mail or teleconferencing. The consumer will do a lot more of his own doctoring. By wearing a "health watch," he will keep a continuous medical

check on his physical and mental state. The data will be fed direct to the computer. Individuals' medical records will be stored in two ways: in a database accessible to anybody with the right password, and on a smart card that is held by the individual.

The computer/doctor will diagnose whatever is wrong with the patient and determine the best treatment. By matching a personal medical profile to databases and services that are available globally, a computer/doctor will be able to tailor advice to patients' needs. If drugs are prescribed, these will be ordered electronically and then mailed to the home; or by using the smart card, they will be obtained from an automatic dispensing machine rather like bank cash machines. At home, online pharmacists or drug manufacturers will be able to advise about therapies.

If surgery is needed, a patient will not need to go to a hospital and stay there. The rapidity with which patients will recover from new surgical procedures will mean that most operations can be performed in a day. . . . [M]any operations will be performed by robots assisted by nurses although specialist surgeons will be called upon (via telemedicine) in emergencies or for tests that robots can still not tackle alone.

What will happen to today's infrastructure? Hospitals are likely to empty as traditional surgical wards become largely redundant. Many will close; others will tend only emergency patients or the chronically ill. Doctors' clinics will also be far less busy. The consumer will take far more responsibility for his own care. In return, the availability and quality of medical help will improve as those delivering health care will have a greater interest in ensuring that their treatments are successful.

As the health care switches to computers and information begins to flow freely among doctors, nurses, drug

makers, and patients, the health care market will become
more transparent. The latest bulletins on the prices and
performance of health care deliverers will be available
on information networks for anybody to read, just as
investors keep in touch with stock market prices. So it
will encourage more competitive buying not just by
insurers and governments but also by patients themselves, making doctors and other health care providers
more accountable than ever before. ["The Future of
Medicine," 1994, pp. 15–16].

While this scenario may seem somewhat Pollyannaish, the
trend is moving in the direction described. What the scenario
doesn't take into account is that many Americans do not have
"homes" in the traditional sense, many do not have the education
and other resources to function effectively in the new "electronic
age," many do not have the financial means to access the "electronic" media, and the scenario does not take into account the
massive resistance by health care professionals to the changes
described. In effect, the challenge is in performing the social and
managerial "engineering" required to making new information
technologies work. It is not yet clear whether the newly emerging
organized delivery systems or eventual community health care
management systems are up to this task.

Demographic Changes

The effect of an aging population on the health care system has been
previously discussed and is well documented. Perhaps even more significant is the growing ethnic and economic diversity of the U.S.
population. For example, between 1980 and 1992, there has been a
65 percent increase in the number of Hispanic Americans, a 123 percent increase in the number of Asian Americans, a 16 percent
increase in the number of African Americans, and a 31 percent increase in American Indians and Eskimos (O'Hare, 1992, p. 10).

Overall, minorities increased by 40 percent between 1980 and 1992 compared with a 6 percent growth in the non-Hispanic white population. In some parts of the country such as Los Angeles, Spanish is spoken by as many people as English. This growing demographic diversity will place new demands on health care delivery systems to meet different cultural definitions of health and illness, different care-seeking behaviors, and different needs and expectations. Greater demands will be placed on viewing the world from the consumers' eyes, taking into account family and community concerns. There will be increased need for culturally sensitive bilingual health care professionals and caregivers able to integrate allopathic and naturopathic healing with Western medicine.

Accompanying the growing demographic diversity will be increases in poverty. Whereas 9 percent of whites were living in poverty in 1991, the figure for African Americans was 33 percent, for Asians 14 percent, for American Indians 32 percent, and for Hispanics 29 percent. The respective percentages for those living in deep poverty (below 50 percent of the official poverty threshold) were 3 percent for whites, 16 percent for African Americans, 7 percent for Asians, 14 percent for American Indians, and 10 percent for Hispanics (O'Hare, 1992, p. 38). Short of major changes in the U.S. economy and social and welfare policy, these figures are not likely to improve. Given the association between income and health status, this means that a growing number of poorer Americans will place additional demands on the health care system. This will be true with or without expansion of health insurance coverage. The net result is that growing ethnic diversity and associated increases in poverty will present major challenges to the ability of organized delivery systems to provide more integrated care.

Restructured Work Force

New technology, changing demographics, a growing emphasis on providing care across the continuum, changes in the education of health care professionals, and new developments in professional licensure and certification result in a host of work force issues facing organized delivery systems. The changes will affect medicine, nursing, pharmacy, and most of the allied health professions.

In medicine, there will be a growing demand for more physicians trained in primary care and less demand for those trained in specialist care. Even within specialist training, greater emphasis will be given to first providing a basis of primary care skills. Lifelong training opportunities will be available for subspecialty internists, obstetricians, and pediatricians to broaden their skills and orientation in becoming primary care generalists. The net result will be a front line of physician providers who are more multiskilled and flexible in meeting patient needs than they are today. At the same time, there will be continued growth in the use of physician assistants and nurse practitioners who will assume expanded roles not only in disease prevention and health promotion but also in helping to manage chronic illness. Most significant, as organized delivery systems continue to evolve, more training will take place at delivery sites that embrace the continuum of care from ambulatory surgery centers, to primary care clinics, to the home.

The impact on nursing may be even more dramatic than the impact on medicine. As more care is provided outside the hospital, there will be a significant reduction in the size of hospital nursing staff, perhaps by as much as 30 percent (O'Neil, 1993). Those remaining will be caring for a very sick group of patients for a shorter period of time. Great demand will be placed on hospital-based nurses to prepare patients and their families for early discharge and for helping to coordinate care with post-hospital caregivers. Some hospital-based nurses will be asked to accompany the patient home and to work with home health agency nurses as part of an overall case or care management approach. While there will be economic incentives for hospitals to substitute lower-cost licensed practical nurses (LPNs) and nurses aides, hospitals may learn that such substitutions will not meet the challenge of providing more coordinated care for a sicker population of patients (Scheffler and Waitzkin, 1996). The result will be an increased demand for nurses with bachelor's degrees and advanced practice training. This trend will be accelerated by clinical reengineering and total quality management efforts, which will identify functions currently performed by allied health professionals (for example, physical therapists, phlebotomists, and so on) that can be performed by nurses with additional training. Finally, there will be an increased demand for nurses who can practice in settings across the continuum of care.

A wide variety of other health professional groups will also be affected. These include pharmacists, physical therapists, occupational therapists, social workers, and various technicians and technologists. As an example, pharmacists will begin to move away from inpatient care toward working on cross-functional teams associated with service lines that care for patients across the continuum. Accompanying this development will be a significant decline in the need for the retail-based pharmacist. As pharmacological agents to prevent and treat disease continue to proliferate, the new health care delivery team is likely to be a triad: the primary care physician, the nurse, and the pharmacist.

For other health professionals, great emphasis will be placed on developing multiple skills permitting flexible deployment throughout the delivery system. The right of any particular group to declare a skill "exclusive" to itself may diminish, and greater attention may be given to licensing the procedure or the skill to be performed than to licensing a given professional group to be the exclusive provider of that skill. If a person can demonstrate competency in the procedure or skill, regardless of their professional degree, they may be allowed to provide the procedure or skill. In some cases, licensure or certification may be granted to the organized delivery system itself, with reliance placed on total quality management, cost-effectiveness, and outcome measures to ensure accountability for quality.

Experimentation may also occur around developing whole new categories of multitrained health professionals, combining basic skills in disease prevention, health education, selected patient treatment techniques and patient monitoring, evaluation, and follow-up. These might be divided into two or three levels such as health professional I, health professional II, and health professional III, based on the level of skill and knowledge required. Each person within each level might then be required to select an "area of concentration" such as physical therapy, occupational therapy, or social work in which they would have some specialized skills.

Health professionals working in public health settings will also be affected by these changes. As organized delivery systems grow, there may be less need for public health professionals to provide direct clinical services. But there will be growing demand for public health professionals with epidemiological and community health status assessment skills and with the ability to work collaboratively with professionals associated with organized delivery systems in addressing community-wide health issues.

In addition to the issues discussed above, there are some education and training initiatives that are likely to be undertaken to help prepare all members of the health care professional work force to practice more effectively within the context of organized delivery systems. Examples include training all health care professionals—physicians, nurses, other caregivers, and future health care executives—in CQI/TQM, in basic epidemiological and community health status assessment skills, and in patient and community outcome assessment methodologies. Efforts to do so are already underway at Dartmouth and several other medical schools. Further, CQI/TQM content, epidemiological content, and team-building content are required in accredited graduate programs in health services administration. Experience suggests that such content can be effectively taught in five-week modules or incorporated within existing courses without eliminating other valued content in the curriculum. In fact, these skills are best taught using experiential exercises in which students work together in teams to solve quality problems or plan services for defined population groups. The bottom line is that a restructured delivery system will require a restructured work force. Our present organized delivery systems are bearing the burden and investment as they find they have to "reengineer" people before they can reengineer and restructure their care processes. To the extent that the health professional schools step up to the challenges outlined above, the task of providing more integrated health care becomes somewhat more manageable.

The likely work force changes we have described will be greatly influenced by continuing technological advances and the overall political context of health care delivery. New technology tends to create greater demand for specialization. This factor will serve as a continual challenge for those attempting to provide multiskilled training designed to promote coordination and integration. The state of the economy will influence the demand and supply of nurses and related health professionals, which will have a ripple effect on who provides what services. Further, the unionization of nurses and other health professionals represents an additional consideration and, in some cases, may serve as a constraint to the ability to re-structure care.

The Demand for Value

We defined *value* in Chapter Three as a relationship between quality attributes desired by consumers and the price consumers must pay to obtain those attributes. Value is created when for a given price to the purchaser, the business provides attributes of service or technical quality that the purchaser desires, and does so in a manner that differentiates itself from competitors. Conversely, value is also created when for a given constellation of quality and service attributes, a lower price can be offered to the purchaser than that of competitors. In the United States we are beginning to question what we are getting for our investment from a value perspective. Higher unit costs explain virtually all of the difference between cost in the United States and that in other countries (Drake, 1994). We practice a more technological, intensive style of medicine and rely more on specialists than do other developed nations. Our unit cost per hospital bed ($170,196) is 62 percent higher than that of the next highest country, Canada (Drake, 1994, p. 139). Paradoxically, technology together with the new private and public managed care pressures provide some of the means and incentives for moving toward a restructured delivery system that promotes equivalent or better outcomes for potentially less cost. A critical question is whether organized delivery systems can respond to the managed care pressures, harness the new technologies, restructure care processes, improve quality and value, and develop outcome reporting and monitoring systems that can document that improvement.

The Role of Organized Delivery Systems

Organized delivery systems can play a major role in dealing with the five driving forces we have outlined—technological change, the information explosion, demographic shifts, a restructured work force, and the growing demand for value. They can do so by channeling these forces in ways that will promote more integrated care of patients in communities rather than fragmented care. Whether or not they will succeed depends largely on the extent to which they can apply the lessons of this book. In brief, they need the necessary vision, leadership, and strategies to drive functional integration, to achieve the requisite level of physician-system integration, and, most important, to make significant progress in the area of clinical integration. As noted, this will require new ways of thinking about health care, new ways of thinking about community, and new management and governance structures. It is of interest to note that the systems in the current study that were further along in their integration efforts were *much less threatened* by state and local health reform and regulatory initiatives than those systems that were less far along. In fact, the systems that were further along were *actively pushing* some of the changes. Thus, the central theses going forward are that organized delivery systems (1) will be in a better position to assess new technologies and be better positioned to diffuse new technologies effectively; (2) will be better able to deal with the information explosion by converting data into information, information into knowledge, and knowledge into wisdom; (3) will better understand and adapt to the demographic changes occurring in society and in their communities and will be better able to serve a diverse consumer base; (4) will be active promoters of a restructured health professional work force that can provide more integrated care across the continuum; and (5) will better understand the new health care value chain and how to best add value along that chain.

As previously noted, organized delivery systems will take many different forms, ranging from tight asset ownership models to looser network models to strategic alliances based on contractual arrangements around a focused set of mutual interests. Current estimates suggest that by the year 2000, standard metropolitan statistical areas (SMSAs) under 450,000 population will average 2 networks; those between 450,000 and one million population will average 3.5 networks; and those with populations over one million will average 5 networks, resulting in a total of 834 networks across 321 SMSAs for an average of about 2.8 networks per SMSA (Weil, 1994). This is generally consistent with existing data suggesting that most markets will have three to four major systems (Luke, 1994). But no one knows which type of model—owned system, affiliated network, strategic alliance, or the many variations of these—will prove most viable and provide the most value in different markets and communities across the United States. However, the research upon which this book is based suggests the critical success factors (discussed in Chapters Four through Seven) that *any* model or approach will need to address. These factors may be thought of as DNA or "organizational code" material for integrated delivery. They may exist in many different structural forms, but if one or more is missing, there will be an "outbreak" of fragmentation within the health care community.

Should Public Policy Encourage Organized Delivery Systems?

"ISNs [integrated service networks] are an organizational black box in which few have looked closely" (Brown, 1994, p. 12). Our present look at one variety of an ISN—namely organized delivery systems—reveals many of the difficulties and challenges to delivering more cost-effective integrated care. Many would agree that the study systems are among some of the leading systems in the nation and are certainly among the most successful performers in the markets in which they are located. Yet their scores on physician-system integration and clinical integration are low, and progress is relatively slow. If this is true for some of the leading organizations, how much more so for those less advanced? Thus the question arises that if there may be some benefits to the formation of such systems, should public policy be enacted to ensure and accelerate their formation and development, and, if so, what should those policies be? Such polices can be categorized into two groups: those that remove current barriers to forming such systems, and those that actively promote or provide incentives for forming such systems.

Removing Barriers

Two primary barriers that require attention are antitrust legislation and personnel licensure and certification.

Antitrust Legislation

Among the most frequently mentioned barriers to system integration is antitrust legislation designed to protect the public from anticompetitive practices that may result from merger and consolidation of organizations (Entin, 1994). The issue is relevant not only to the consolidation or merger of hospitals but also to physicians' ability to organize themselves into various groups and networks and to enter into arrangements with hospitals and health systems (Padden, 1995). In response, some states, such as Maine, Minnesota, Ohio, Washington, and Wisconsin, have enacted hospital cooperation laws that allow providers to enter into cooperative arrangements with each other if the likely benefits to the community outweigh the potential disadvantages due to a reduction in competition (Blumstein, 1994; Felsenthal, 1993; Iglehart, 1993). Prudent policy would suggest that hospitals and other health care providers not be totally exempted from the antitrust laws but rather that there be greater flexibility in application, a greater understanding of the intent and operation of the organizations and providers coming together to form integrated delivery, and a broad consideration of potential benefits to the community. There is also need to recognize that assessments of the benefits and threats of organized delivery systems to the community are different from assessments based on considerations of individual hospitals. It may that the issue has been given more attention than it deserves: a recent review of 397 hospital mergers indicates that 83 percent have been allowed to proceed without further inquiry, 13 percent were cleared after further investigations, and only 4 percent were directly challenged (U.S. General Accounting Office, 1995). Nonetheless, as the health care industry goes through third- and fourth-wave "partnering" activity, anticompetitive concerns are likely to heighten, and the need for informed and flexible antitrust policies will be critical (Zelman, 1995).

Personnel Licensure and Certification

A key aspect of providing more integrated health care is the ability to use multiskilled professionals in a flexible fashion. Nurses can be trained to take on some of the functions of other professionals, such as physical therapists and phlebotomists, and some of these other groups can be trained to take on additional responsibilities as well. Reflecting this need, entirely new categories of health workers are being created such as *patient support attendants* who perform the functions of housekeeping, dietary, transportation, and materials management; *patient care technicians* who perform phlebotomies, ECGs, selected respiratory therapy tasks, selected rehab tasks, and related nursing assistant tasks; *acute care RN case managers* who plan and coordinate in-hospital care for selected groups of patients; and *primary care RN case managers* who perform similar responsibilities for patients receiving care outside the hospital setting (Parsons, 1995). Yet many systems are restricted in their ability to use professionals in more flexible ways by licensing and certification laws—often, of course, designed by the professionals themselves to protect their job and sense of professional identity. But as cost-containment pressures intensify, resulting in the potential for direct job loss, many of these same professionals are becoming more open to job expansion, retraining, and the creation of new roles. There is need for legislative experimentation to promote such flexibility, with greater consideration given to institutional licensure that relies on patient outcome and satisfaction measures for accountability. In certain procedural areas involving a high degree of technical skill, licensure or certification bodies could require a number of procedures to be performed under supervision and a set number of hours of continuing education to be completed by the health professional performing the procedure, regardless of his or her degree or particular health care profession. As patient care restructuring continues to evolve and as CQI/TQM activities are used to assist organizations in their search for more cost-effective ways to deliver care, new roles and responsibilities will emerge that can only be roughly foreseen at present. A new set of competencies and accountability criteria must be developed that facilitate these innovations.

Providing Incentives

A number of incentives involving financial issues, benefit packages, new types of health professionals, and group practice formation should be considered.

Common Financial Incentives

As long as different components of the system face different economic incentives, efforts to cooperate in providing a more coordinated array of services across the continuum of care will be severely compromised. One of the most pervasive complaints of those interviewed in the Health Systems Integration Study pertained to the mixed financial incentives created by the mix of indemnity-based fee-for-service payment, discounted fee for service, partial capitation, and full capitation arrangements (Shortell, Gillies, and Anderson, 1994). The greatest potential for creating shared economic incentives lies in the development of capitated payment or budgets that embrace all components of care—physicians, ambulatory surgery centers, home health, hospitals, long-term care, and so on. Full capitation places all providers in the delivery chain at risk and provides incentives for them to work together in cost-effective ways to earn the residual between the money spent and the predetermined revenue limit. It also provides incentives for providers to place greater emphasis on disease prevention, health maintenance, and health promotion. There is also suggestive evidence from the study (using the measures described in Chapter Six) that systems operating under a high degree of capitated payment are further along in their clinical integration efforts (Shortell, Gillies, and Anderson, 1994). As others have emphasized, payment and delivery are intertwined (Jones and Mayerhofer, 1994). It is not possible to achieve greater integration of care in local communities without common economic incentives. Fragmented payment leads to fragmented delivery.

A major issue in this regard is that capitation is generally not available for the self-insured employer. The current regulatory environment in many states allows self-insured employers to utilize the discounted fee schedules of a PPO network or those offered by an organized delivery system but generally does not allow the employer to transfer utilization risk (insurance or actuarial risk) through capitation or other forms of withhold arrangements. Without some form of risk transference to or risk sharing with the organized delivery system, however, the traditional incentives to provide more health care than is clinically necessary would remain unchanged.

This scenario has played out in Minneapolis and St. Paul where a large coalition of self-insured businesses—the Buyer's Health Care Action Group (BHCAG)—selected a provider network organized by the Group Care Consortium for its preferred delivery system in 1993. Because of the regulations described above, BHCAG had to create a fee schedule by which its provider payments would be determined. Knowing this payment mechanism lacked the incentives necessary to encourage appropriate provider behaviors, BHCAG chose a provider system that had historically functioned under capitation. Both the employers and the providers have recognized the need for "capitation-like" incentives and are looking to restructure their future financial arrangement.

An argument could be made that the Employee Retirement Income Security Act (ERISA) of 1974, as amended, preempts the regulation of an organized delivery system that contracts with a self-insured employer. Therefore, the self-insured employer could develop unique payment relationships with providers and not be subject to a state's regulations for insurance.

With a substantial portion of the United States work force covered by self-insured employers, the regulatory environment should promote incentives for less fragmented and more cost-effective health care.

Providing a Coordinated Benefit Package

Carved out benefits—whether for mental health, long-term care, or cancer care—are inimical to integration. They lead to the establishment of separate delivery and administrative mechanisms, creating coordination problems within local communities. Although the costs will be higher, health benefit packages must be reasonably comprehensive in order to assure that care will be coordinated across the continuum. If benefits such as mental health, substance abuse, and various components of long-term care are left uncovered, these services will essentially be uncoordinated with other aspects of the delivery system. Policy makers need to realize that the issues of carve outs and restricted benefits will grow in importance as the number of individuals experiencing multiple chronic illnesses increases. A seventy-five-year-old diabetic suffering from cancer and heart disease may have *three* sets of "carved out" benefits, with each potentially involving a different delivery system. Benefit design exerts as much influence on service delivery as do the payment incentives noted above. In brief, payment, benefit design, and delivery system organization must be aligned for patients to receive maximum value.

Producing New Types of Health Professionals

Given the need for a restructured work force as previously described, there is need for radical changes in health professional education. It is estimated that 75 percent of HMOs believe internists are not well prepared to manage care; 62 percent of HMOs report that pediatricians are not well prepared (Zelman, 1995, p. 103). Change is needed in both the *types* of professionals produced as well as *how* and where they are taught. Although the need for a greater number of primary care physicians may be somewhat less than originally thought, there is clearly a need for fewer physicians in most specialties and subspecialties. For example, a recent Council of Graduate Medical Education report predicts an excess of 115,000 specialists by the year 2000 (Zelman, 1995, p. 103). As more care is provided in outpatient, home, and work settings, there is also a need to reexamine the numbers and types of all health professionals that will be required. There may well be a need for fewer physicians but more nurses, physician assistants, social workers, and perhaps whole new categories of multidisciplinary, multiskilled professionals that might be called patient care coordinators, patient care technicians, or community health care managers.

Perhaps even more important than the types of providers needed is how they will need to be educated and trained. There is need for marked change in content to incorporate CQI/TQM into the curricula for all health care professionals. Greater emphasis must be given to working in teams, to basic data analysis skills, to clinical epidemiology, to clinical decision analysis, to development of protocols and pathways, and to use of patient outcome and community health status assessment instruments. As previously noted, this need not require separate or additional courses but with imagination can be incorporated into existing courses and, in particular, into internship and residency programs. Of particular note is the need for all those aspiring to be health professionals to have a mental model of what constitutes a healthy community; of what produces, maintains, and enhances health; of where the key breakdowns lie; and then determine what kinds of interventions and follow-up processes are most likely to lead to effective restoration of health or amelioration of the illness or disease. Health professionals may each be responsible for only a small portion of the continuum of care, but they must see the big picture and recognize the inherent interdependence of their work with that of others. Most important, health professionals must be taught skills that empower the community and patients to recognize that they bear the primary responsibility for their health, and that when illness strikes, they must be intimately involved in all aspects of their care.

Promoting Group Practice

As discussed in Chapter Five, physicians practicing in groups are an important component of physician-system integration, which is in turn strongly associated with clinical integration. While the percentage of physicians practicing in groups is slowly growing, it is highly uneven across the country. Thus, consideration might be given to policies at either the state or national level to stimulate more physicians to join group practices. Several alternatives exist. One would be to provide direct subsidies to physicians or delivery systems to form group practices. Alternatively, low-interest loans could be provided for group practice formation. Still another approach would be to allow systems or physicians who are organized into groups within systems to keep a higher percentage of savings under capitated budgets. These alternatives might best be viewed as jump-start policies, as it is likely that they could be phased out after three or four years once a majority of physicians (for example, 75 percent) are organized into groups of one form or another.

Special Initiatives

State or federal government might also develop legislation that would directly encourage the further growth and development of organized delivery systems. Some aspects of such legislation might include the following: (1) grants and/or loans for network and system development targeted to underdeveloped areas and populations; (2) state licensure of regional health systems based on predetermined access, service, quality, and outcome criteria in return for which the system would be exempt from certificate-of-need legislation, would be freely able to relocate facilities and bed capacity, would be able to reconfigure levels of care, and would be able to use personnel in flexible ways (Jones and Mayerhofer, 1994); (3) "reverse" Hill-Burton legislation to buy and close unneeded facilities by retiring debt and assuming other liabilities (Jones and Mayerhofer, 1994); (4) exemption from corporate practice of medicine laws (applicable in California, Texas, and four other states); (5) exemption from Stark anti-referral legislation; (6) exemption from any-willing-provider legislation; (7) where a delivery system accepts risk, protection from state laws that regulate insurers; and (8) flexibility in regard to capital insolvency requirements in recognition that an organized delivery system may not have the same strict capital reserve requirements of a traditional indemnity insurance carrier.

The Downside of Encouraging Organized Delivery Systems

While this book has emphasized the potential of organized delivery systems to overcome the fragmentation in health care delivery, and presented some evidence to support this potential, it is important to recognize that the evidence is in the early formative stage. It may well be likened to a phase one or, at best, phase two clinical trial still awaiting the more definitive phase three findings. An argument can thus be made that we should simply wait and see. If the organized delivery system concept "holds water," then natural market forces should operate to encourage its expansion with no need for special policy initiatives.

Arguments can also be made that organized delivery systems may actually have negative consequences. Aside from the antitrust issues of monopoly and oligopoly power, there is the concern that organized delivery systems will "take care of their own" but not truly reach across the community to serve those with the most serious health problems. For example, will organized delivery systems really provide an integrated continuum of care for the disabled, the mentally ill, or those suffering from substance abuse or Alzheimer's disease? A related concern is that they may actually displace organizations (public institutions and neighborhood health centers, for example) currently caring for the poor, the disadvantaged, and those with multiple chronic illnesses (Brown, 1994). There are also concerns regarding the dysfunctional consequences of large size, namely increased bureaucracy and a diminished ability to respond to changing consumer needs. Finally, there is skepticism that the large national systems and chains, whether for-profit or not-for-profit, may be too far removed from local communities to effectively address local needs. But whether or not policy should be enacted to actively encourage organized delivery systems, the issue of how best to hold such systems accountable is an immediate issue.

How Should Organized Delivery Systems Be Held Accountable?

Organized delivery systems present both problems and new opportunities regarding notions of accountability. A major issue involves fixing the *scope* of accountability. Clearly such systems can and will be held accountable for their "enrolled lives"—the people who choose the system and pay the capitated dollars. Many systems, faithful to their mission of serving the poor, will also provide care to those in their own geographic area and will be held accountable by their community-oriented boards. But there are also opportunities for such systems to be held responsible for the overall health status of the larger community they serve—particularly with systems' emphasis on prevention, wellness, and more integrated care. At the same time, however, overlapping boundaries among systems in a given area may make it difficult to fix accountability. Further, some of the health status indicators may be influenced by events not under the systems' control. It is in this latter area that organized delivery systems must work with each other and with public health and social service agencies, schools, law enforcement agencies, and work sites to influence community health. This is an extremely difficult process involving different social contexts, different financial incentives and resources, and different cultures, even if one can achieve agreement on goals. McKnight (1992) has noted that health systems and communities are different tools to do different work. Health systems essentially repair illness and disease through the use of professional expertise and power. Communities rely on shared collective wisdom and widespread participation to attack complex and intertwined "wicked" problems— problems that often defy accurate description or definition. To help bridge the gap, health systems must respect citizen input, appreciate diversity, share information in understandable forms, use their skills and resources to strengthen local groups, and be willing to be "servant organizations" that empower others to assume the leadership role. The new expertise of such health systems will lie in the ability to empower the communities in which they reside (Bethell, 1995).

While this represents an ideal, there are some more near-term accountability issues that must be addressed. At what level(s) should accountability be placed, and what criteria should be used to hold delivery systems accountable? Among the options are state commissioners of health, state-appointed health councils (or similar bodies), local or regional community health councils or boards, and permutations of the above. Minnesota has taken the first approach, whereby integrated service networks would be held accountable on various criteria (quality and outcomes of care, service availability, and so on) to the state health commissioner. Washington State proposed to create statewide health care authorities or boards to oversee delivery system reform and the performance of health plans and organized delivery systems, although electoral changes threaten full implementation. Others argue that the most appropriate place to fix accountability is locally within communities and regions that are closest to the issues (Sigmond, 1995). For example, the Jewish Health Care Foundation of Pittsburgh has proposed development of a *local health assurance organization* to promote the formation of integrated health systems and to hold them accountable (Jewish Healthcare Foundation, 1995). The agency would help develop a consensus vision on comprehensive care for the community and monitor the effectiveness of systems in achieving those objectives by issuing periodic report cards. They would also conduct studies on issues of special importance. They would require an expert staff to help carry out the analytic functions, working collaboratively with local universities and research institutes. A major issue posed by such community-based groups is the relationship between them and statewide health care bodies. Ultimately, the local group would require delegated powers from the state to monitor and evaluate performance in order to have any lasting influence. Figure 8.1 provides a further description of how such a system might operate.

The list that follows provides a set of shared values that might be embraced.

*Shared Community Values to Guide the Evolution
of a Reformed Health Care System*

- Individuals are responsible for maintaining their health, with help from their communities and the health care system.

- A comprehensive health system is responsible for the health of both the individuals and the population in its community.

- Health status assessment is an ongoing responsibility of the health system. Prevention programs depend on these studies.

- Out of fairness, insurance coverage should be universal with a standard benefit package and

Figure 8.1. Health Assurance Corporation Function Chart.

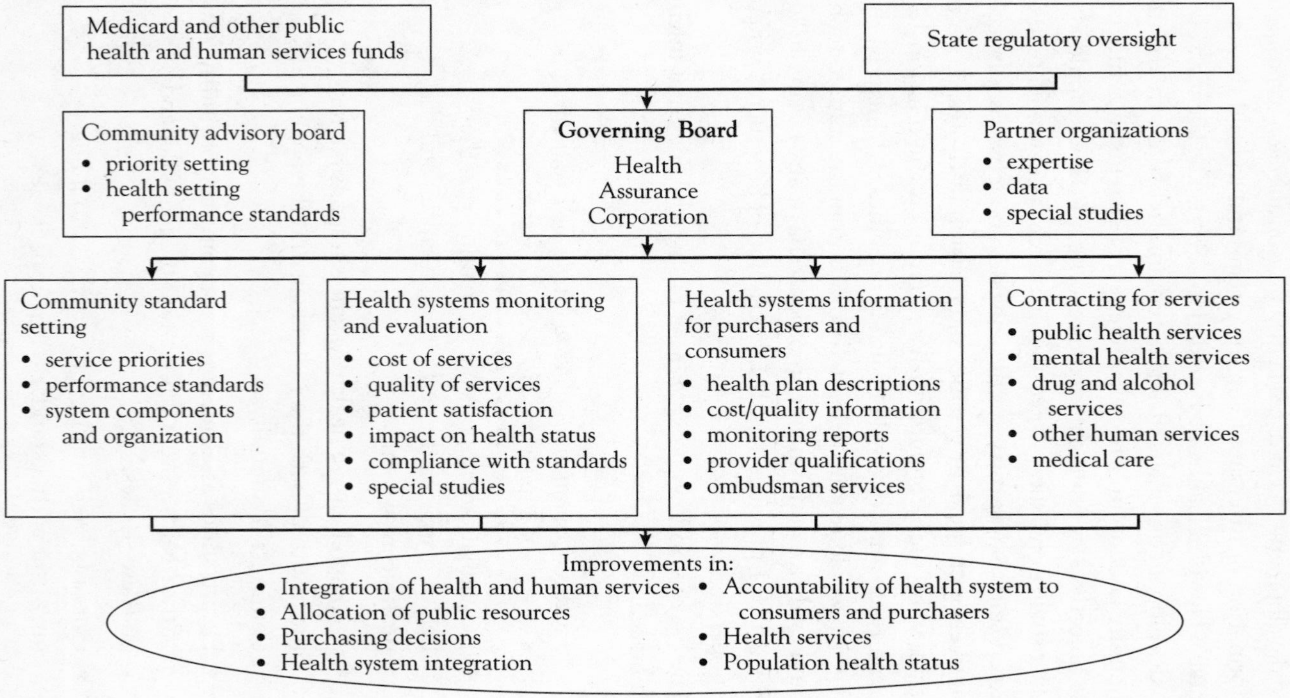

Medicard and other public
health and human services funds

State regulatory oversight

Community advisory board
- priority setting
- health setting
- performance standards

Governing Board

Health
Assurance
Corporation

Partner organizations
- expertise
- data
- special studies

Community standard
setting
- service priorities
- performance standards
- system components
  and organization

Health systems monitoring
and evaluation
- cost of services
- quality of services
- patient satisfaction
- impact on health status
- compliance with standards
- special studies

Health systems information
for purchasers and
consumers
- health plan descriptions
- cost/quality information
- monitoring reports
- provider qualifications
- ombudsman services

Contracting for services
- public health services
- mental health services
- drug and alcohol
  services
- other human services
- medical care

Improvements in:
- Integration of health and human services
- Allocation of public resources
- Purchasing decisions
- Health system integration
- Accountability of health system to
  consumers and purchasers
- Health services
- Population health status

Source: "Health Environmental Scan," *Jewish Healthcare Foundation,* 1995, p. 25. Reprinted with permission of the publisher.

community-rated premiums. It should be portable
between jobs and be subsidized when necessary.

- Everyone should have a responsible health care
  provider.

- Most people place a high value on selecting their
  own health services providers.

- Health services should be convenient, timely, coordinated, dignified, culturally acceptable, and easy
  to use.

- The poor and other vulnerable populations require
  special provisions to facilitate best use of health services.

- Realistic limitations on medical care may be necessary to restrain costs.

- The community has a legitimate interest in guiding
  the evolution of the health system. Health care
  providers must be accountable to the consumers and
  purchasers of care. ["Health Environmental Scan,"
  1995, p. 23]

A second issue involves the criteria for accountability. There is
always the temptation to develop a comprehensive set of criteria
that may make sense conceptually but may be difficult or impossible to implement. This is particularly true in regard to outcome
measures, given the current status of clinical information systems
and, indeed, knowledge of cause and effect relationships in health
care delivery. A productive approach might be to use the concept
of a balanced portfolio of accountability measures or what some
have called "balanced scorecards" (Kaplan and Norton, 1993), an
example of which is provided by the Henry Ford Health System in
Chapter Six. These would include a variety of licensing standards,
access criteria, service availability criteria, cost, quality, outcomes
(where available), and information sharing requirements. Financial

criteria might include cost per enrolled member adjusted for health status; access criteria might include the percentage of people below or near the poverty line that are cared for; quality criteria might include the provision of care consistent with guidelines, protocols, and pathways for selected conditions; and outcome criteria might include risk-adjusted mortality for selected conditions, readmission rates for selected conditions, functional health status scores, and patient satisfaction ratings.

As organized delivery systems take on direct risks, or as purchasers contract directly with delivery systems, accountability criteria must be developed that take into account how organized delivery systems are different from traditional insurers ("Hospitals, Integrated Delivery Systems," 1995; Zelman, 1995). Relevant issues involve capital requirements, provider credentialing, quality assessment and improvement criteria, utilization review, confidentiality, and data reporting.

A number of states are in the process of developing such accountability standards for organized delivery systems. For example, Minnesota requires integrated service networks to provide a comprehensive range of services, to enroll high-risk subscribers, to prohibit dropping people from plans because of illness or risk, and to provide clear, understandable marketing information to potential subscribers. California has recently passed legislation requiring hospitals to do a community needs assessment and file a community benefits plan with a statewide office of health planning and development (1994 Cal ALS 812, 1994). The assessment must include a process for consulting with community groups and local officials. It must be updated every three years and a report made on effectiveness in achieving the plan's objectives. Examples of other requirements might be to require organized delivery systems to participate in Medicare and Medicaid experiments, to work out linkages with rural providers where relevant, and to work with public health and community service agencies in developing programs for such targeted problems and diseases as AIDS, smoking, and traffic accidents. Washington State, for example, is in the process of developing a Public Health Improvement Plan targeted to such problems as AIDS, tobacco use, infant mortality, and hazardous substances (Alpha Center, 1995).

Some Special Issues

The challenges of overcoming fragmentation to achieve more cost-effective integrated delivery of health services raise special issues for academic medical centers, vulnerable populations, and residents of rural America. Each of these are highlighted below along with some suggestions for dealing with the challenges.

The Academic Medical Center

Perhaps no institution will be more affected by the changes occurring in health care than teaching hospitals associated with academic medical centers. These institutions are getting hit from all sides simultaneously. On the patient care delivery side, they are subject to the same managed care pressures to reduce costs as everyone else (Fox and Wasserman, 1993). On the teaching side, they are being asked to devote more of their patient care earnings to support medical education at a time in which payers do not wish to pay for these costs. Further, there are proposals to limit payment for residents in certain specialties in order to address manpower imbalances. But residents are also a relatively inexpensive form of labor for teaching hospitals. On the research front, the costs of doing research are growing at a time when NIH funding is declining. At the same time, many teaching hospitals associated with academic medical centers, particularly those located in the inner city, provide a disproportionate share of care for the medically indigent. These hospitals also face stiff competition from surrounding suburban community hospitals that are often able to offer essentially the same treatment technology at a lower cost because they do not have the same degree of teaching and research commitments as the academic teaching hospital. Many of the suburban physicians have in fact been trained by the local academic medical center that has, in effect, created its own competition. The situation is aptly summarized by Bob Baker, president of the University Hospital Consortium, which represents sixty-seven of the major teaching hospitals across the United States: "There is no way academic medical centers will be able to cover their education and research costs without a stable source of support that replaces their reduced ability to cross-subsidize. These developments are compelling academic centers to lower their costs and consider seriously downsizing their hospitals and clinical and support staffs if they are going to successfully weather these fundamental changes in the health care system" (Iglehart, 1995, p. 407).

While there is need for more efficient ways of conducting teaching and research activities, the immediate challenge facing these hospitals is to redesign the way in which they provide care. Some progress is being made, as evidenced by cost reductions of between $29 million and $75 million in one year on the part of some teaching hospitals (Cochrane, 1995). But this is the easy stuff. The really difficult task for academic medical centers is to create a more integrated delivery system that can address patient needs across the continuum of care. The integration challenge is both internal and external.

Academic medical centers must first get their internal houses in order. There are strong internal barriers, including different organizational structures, incentives, cultures, and goals for the hospital, the faculty practice plan, and the medical school. In addition, within the faculty practice plan, numerous fiefdoms are organized around departmental and subspecialty interests. In recent years, some medical schools, such as at Emory, Johns Hopkins, Illinois, Massachusetts, Minnesota, and Stanford, have attempted to integrate the three entities based on more shared management and governance structures linked by a common strategic planning process.

A recent report by the University Hospital Consortium has underscored the need for all academic medical centers to develop a "more integrated clinical enterprise" (Hart, 1995, p. 409). The barriers, however, are formidable, as department chairs fight to protect valued interests and the different entities—hospital, faculty practice plan, and medical school—struggle to find the intersecting space in a Venn diagram where these interests might coincide.

Dealing with the internal issues only means that the academic medical center can play in the game. They then must develop a coherent strategy for dealing with all of the rapidly changing forces stimulated by managed care pressures. One big decision is whether to join a network or system or to develop one of their own. This, of course, will vary depending on the strength and cultural compatibility of existing networks or systems within a given market, the intensity of managed care pressure within the market, and the degree of leadership and "managed care readiness" on the part of the academic medical center itself. Brigham and Women's Hospital and Massachusetts General Hospital in Boston, Johns Hopkins in Baltimore, Northwestern Memorial Hospital in Chicago, University of California Medical Center in San Diego, and Stanford in Palo Alto are all examples of academic medical centers that have decided to form their own networks or systems, often with surrounding community hospitals.

A second major decision involves developing a specific primary care strategy for competing in the managed care environment. Among the options are to use the faculty practice plan as the core primary care base, to purchase primary care practices directly or create a joint venture with a partner, or to pursue strategic alliances with community-based primary care physicians. Again, depending on market conditions and each organization's capabilities, there are pros and cons to each approach. Many academic medical centers are pursuing all three strategies simultaneously. Pursuing a faculty practice plan strategy alone probably entails the most risk because these plans have a strong specialist base and little interest in expanding into primary care. The primary care groups within the faculty practice plan often cannot compete on a cost basis with community-based groups. This often necessitates buying physician practices. This represents a cornerstone of University of Pennsylvania's $100 million strategy to develop an external primary care network throughout the greater Philadelphia area (Iglehart, 1995, p. 410). Others, such as Duke and Tulane, are finding "deep pocket" partners with which to create joint ventures in purchasing and managing physician practices. In areas where a substantial base of primary care already exists, various arrangements are being made with community-based primary care physicians. The academic medical center typically agrees to provide practice support and, in some cases, expand involvement of community physicians in the teaching and clinical research activities of the academic medical center.

By far the biggest challenge academic medical centers will face is *cultural*. If the U.S. health care system has a general problem with fragmentation, academic medical centers have a full-blown epidemic of the "disease." The role of the academic medical center has been to push the limits of science and develop new diagnostic and treatment technologies—most of which until recently have been used in acute inpatient care. Because of this, making the transition from the "hospital as hub" to the "hospital as periphery" of the health system is particularly difficult. Academic medical centers are very good at high-tech inpatient care, but they are not very good at delivering low-tech primary care. Commitments to teaching and research complicate this transition process. And, most significant, many of those physicians and other health professionals associated with academic medical centers have views of what constitutes "quality of care" that are quite different from those operating in a managed care environment. As expressed by one academic medical center physician: "They are asking us to provide GEO Prizm care when we are used to providing a Lexus. Maybe we have to create different product lines. But I still want to be associated with a Lexus." At least this physician recognizes the need for a more cost-effective "product line." The next challenge will come when he learns that there may not be enough money to produce the Lexus anymore and that most of the capitated dollars in the budget are going into expansion of the GEO Prizm line.

Our present study suggests that those academic medical centers that understand the building blocks of integration and that develop the capabilities to construct them will succeed. Many will not be able to do this on their own and will thus benefit greatly from linking with existing systems and networks that can help accelerate the learning process.

Serving Vulnerable Populations

Vulnerable populations are those at risk for illness, disease, and/or injury and without the ability for financial or other reasons to receive the needed care. The question is whether organized delivery systems will be better able to deal with these groups than are other approaches to care. From our experience, the answer is yes, if there is a real commitment to do so.

In *Mama Would Be Better Off Dead* (Abraham, 1994), a Chicago-area reporter documents the experience of the Banes family in their attempt to receive medical care for various diseases over a one-year period. Despite the well-intentioned efforts of many people, there are numerous examples of delayed and missed appointments, lack of communication, incorrect treatment, and lack of follow-up care. A few brief excerpts are of interest:

> It is not unusual for physicians to have only cursory involvement of home health patients at Mt. Sinai and elsewhere. (p. 70)
>
> Irregular primary care had been a problem for Mrs. Jackson from the start when diabetic gangrene was first diagnosed in her right foot in February. (p. 60)
>
> "I was thinking there wasn't that much wrong. I thought whatever it was might clear up on its own. They

told me I had something of my kidney, but nobody told me to come back" (p. 31)

"Many devices or supplies can prevent disease and disability from worsening. I'm not covered by Medicare because its reimbursement criteria emphasize curing acute conditions rather than maintaining health or improving daily function—a policy that may be penny wise but pound foolish" (p. 48).

The family encountered the usual fragmented delivery system that exists in most metropolitan communities throughout the United States—no better and no worse. An organized delivery system that functions as a truly *clinically integrated* delivery system would have ameliorated many of this family's problems. The most beneficial mechanism probably would have been to assign a *family* health care manager—probably a nurse practitioner—whose responsibility it would be to oversee the interdependent needs of the family members and who would help orchestrate their care by staying in close contact with the several different physicians and other health professionals that the family encountered.

Most of the systems in the study have as an important part of their mission the commitment to serve those in need, including those without the ability to pay. Several systems, primarily those with religious roots, have lost considerable sums of money (for example, $12 million a year) in providing care to the inner-city poor. They continue to remain in those communities and to explore creative strategies for long-run involvement. A number of systems, as previously noted, have also been proactive in working with community leaders on underlying causes of health problems, involving issues of education, jobs, housing, and public safety. But one cannot expect all organized delivery systems to take on such commitments.

A related question is to ask whether such systems will be willing and able to pick up the care provided by public and safety net providers squeezed by Medicaid and Medicare cuts. Will organized delivery systems pick up the slack? Will they be willing to enter into joint ventures with public institutions? As previously mentioned, state and federal initiatives to hold organized delivery systems accountable should contain provisions for treatment of vulnerable populations and incentives to enter into collaborative relationships with current public providers of these services where feasible. If it is the case that organized delivery systems are able to provide a broader range of coordinated, accountable care (than more loosely organized alternatives), then there is a rationale behind government initiatives to encourage organized delivery systems' involvement in addressing problems of vulnerable populations.

Health Care in Rural America

Can organized delivery systems meet the needs of rural America? Is it possible to form such systems in rural America? How should the value chain of clinically integrated health care be put together to serve rural Americans?

In addressing these questions it is important to recognize the diversity of rural America. Some rural communities are relatively contiguous to metropolitan areas; others are extremely remote (for example, large parts of Alaska, Wyoming, Montana, and North and South Dakota) and are often referred to as "frontier" areas (Fickenscher and Lagerwey-Voorman, 1992). It is obviously easier to coordinate a continuum of services in the former case than in the latter. The questions are largely ones of where best to locate services, given the needs and preferences of rural residents, and of how to staff the services.

There are basically three options for rural providers: (1) continue to go it alone, (2) form a rural system or network with other rural institutions, or (3) join with an urban- or suburban-based network or system. It is becoming generally accepted that the first strategy is not viable (Bray and others, 1994). In regard to the second strategy, there are relatively few rural networks that provide a comprehensive array of services (Moscovice, 1994). Those networks that have been developed have proven to be relatively unstable (Moscovice and others, 1995). Among the barriers have been limited capital and technical expertise, physician resistance, lack of leadership, and a shortage of primary care providers. The exceptions are a few organizations such as Geisinger and the Mayo Clinic that have a long history and tradition associated with developing an infrastructure that will support effective delivery of rural health services in a managed care environment.

Perhaps the most viable model will be the linkage of rural institutions with urban- or suburban-based networks and systems, whereby the rural institutions draw on the financial, technical, and organizational resources of these systems. Several of the study systems (Baylor, Fairview, Franciscan, Sisters of Providence, and Sutter) had significant successful linkages with rural areas. Most of the rural institutions were members of regional or subregional components of the overall system and full participants in system management and governance. Intermountain Health Care represents another example of an urban-based (Salt Lake City) health system that has significant rural commitments, throughout Utah, Wyoming, and Idaho. In order to further stimulate such linkages, policies might be enacted that provide incentives for urban-based systems and networks to partner with rural communities through the use of development funds for manpower re-deployment and telecommunications. These policies would need to remain flexible in their application of antitrust laws and would have to recognize the need for modified solvency standards for developing rural-based HMOs.

The New Bottom Line

Speaking optimistically, public policies might be devised that would encourage the integration of medicine, management, and public health with the community (see Figure 8.2).

Figure 8.2. Building the Community Health Care Management System.

Environment

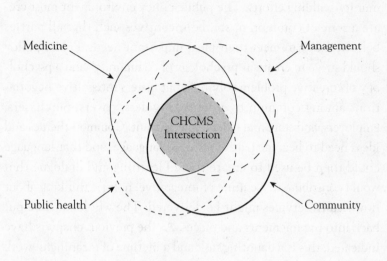

Environment

Realistically, the hope might be that public policies are at least neutral to such integration. Achieving clinically integrated systems of care is difficult enough without having to face an incoherent, contradictory policy and regulatory framework. As Brown cogently notes, "New integrated systems offer no special magic as the [health] system contemplates tradeoffs and conflicts it has dodged for years. Their performance can be no better than the public policy framework within which they operate and evolve." (Brown, 1994, p. 16). The challenge is not confined to the United States. Canada (Leatt, Pink, and Naylor, 1995), Great Britain, Germany, New Zealand, and other nations are all searching for more cost-effective ways to deliver health services and are learning that at least part of the answer lies in establishing incentives that encourage a fundamental reexamination of how to provide patient care.

A major theme of this book, introduced in Chapters One and Two, was the need for community-building. Building organized delivery systems that last will depend on the strength of local community-building efforts. The public policy environment must create a zone of common or shared incentives such that all parties believe they can meet their most important needs. Public policy should strive to create a "psychology of community" and a psychology of "creative problem solving" that fosters integrative negotiations among community groups, providers, payers, purchasers, employers, and state and federal government. Common themes and ideas need to become part of a shared language, and that language could then be used to create shared learning and dialogue that would contribute to a culture of integrative, holistic thinking about how health services might be delivered. The whole must be put back into the fragments and pieces. As the previous chapters have indicated, this is a daunting task and a lifetime of meaningful work for all involved. But, given the money that Americans are currently spending in their love-hate relationship with the health system, it might be worth the effort.

Resource A

About the Study

Advocate Health Care (Formerly EHS Health Care)

•••••••••••••••••••••••••••••••••

EHS Health Care

Headquarters   Oak Brook, Illinois

Area(s) served   Chicago metropolitan area

Total revenues $748.5 million (December 1994)

Total assets $803.2 million (December 1994)

Operating units   Owned five acute care hospitals and one specialty hospital and was affiliated with one other acute care hospital (total of 2,068 licensed acute care beds). Also owned three nursing homes, nine retirement centers, a home health division (included both a not-for-profit agency and a for-profit agency), a diagnostic imaging center, an ambulatory surgery center, and a philanthropic foundation. Had 50 percent ownership in five physician-hospital organizations.

Note: Additional detail for each of the systems is available at cost by contacting: the Health Systems Integration Project, Attn.: Robin Gillies, Ph.D., Health Services Management, Kellogg Graduate School of Management, Leverone Hall, Northwestern University, 2001 Sheridan Road, Evanston, IL 60208–2007.

Managed care Had 50 percent ownership in Health Direct, Inc., a managed care firm with full insurance capability, offering a traditional HMO, a point-of-service HMO, and a PPO to area employers. Also had fifteen direct contracts with employers, covering more than 400,000 people.

Advocate Health Care

Created January 1995 by a merger of EHS Health Care and Lutheran General HealthSystem of Park Ridge, Illinois

Headquarters Oak Brook, Illinois

Area(s) served Greater Chicago metropolitan area; divided into three operating regions (North, South and Central) with a total of 180 sites of care

Total revenues $1.4 billion combined (1994)

Total assets $1.6 billion combined (1994)

Operating units Has six owned and two affiliated hospitals with a total of 3,308 beds; four extended care facilities (675 beds total); and numerous outpatient diagnostic centers and physician office buildings throughout the Chicago area

Managed care Owns Health Direct, Inc., a managed care organization that includes an HMO and a PPO covering a combined total of 336,000 people

Baylor Health Care System

Headquarters Dallas, Texas

Area(s) served Dallas metropolitan area

Total revenues $631.4 million (June 1994)

Total assets $875.2 million (June 1994)

Operating units Has full ownership of five acute care hospitals (total of 1,454 licensed acute care beds), six senior health centers, two specialty hospitals and one of each of the following: PPO, PHO, home health care agency, ambulatory surgery center, sports medicine and research center, and durable medical equipment company. Manages four single-specialty physician group practices.

Managed care Has full ownership in Southwest Preferred Health Network (PPO); minority ownership in Aetna-SWHP (HMO) and North Texas Health Network

Fairview Hospital & Healthcare Services

Headquarters Minneapolis, Minnesota

Area(s) served Twin Cities metropolitan area and areas northeast of the Twin Cities metropolitan area

Total revenues $514.0 million (December 1994)

Total assets $476.2 million (December 1994)

Operating units Owns six general acute care hospitals (with 1,836 total licensed beds), twenty primary care clinics, one skilled nursing facility, one home health agency, one ambulatory surgery center, four retail pharmacies, an offshore insurance captive (one unit), Healthworks (two units), the Institute for Athletic Medicine (twenty-one units), one PHO, and one philanthropic foundation.

Managed care Has 60 percent ownership in a managed care company, which manages a PPO and a long-term contracting relationship with a staff-model HMO (Health Partners).

Franciscan Health System

Headquarters Aston, Pennsylvania

Area(s) served   Mid-Atlantic region (including eastern Pennsylvania, Delaware, Maryland, and New Jersey) and the Pacific Northwest (Oregon and Washington State)

Total revenues $1.0 billion (June 30, 1994)

Total assets $1.0 billion (June 30, 1993)

Operating units   Owns thirteen acute care hospitals (eight in the Eastern region and five in the Western region, with a total of 3,211 licensed acute care beds in the thirteen hospitals), ten nursing homes, one extended care facility, eight home health care agencies, six durable medical equipment companies (some through joint ventures), three diagnostic imaging centers, four ambulatory surgery centers, three hundred employed physicians in three primary care group practices, ten PHOs, ten philanthropic foundations, and a mobile MRI multisite unit.

Managed care   FHS does not have a system-level managed care division. Managed care contracting is handled at the regional level. FHS is evaluating joint venture opportunities and risk contracts with various HMOs in FHS-East and FHS-West markets.

Henry Ford Health System

Headquarters   Detroit, Michigan

Area(s) served   Detroit metropolitan area

Total revenues $1.5 billion (December 1994)

Total assets $1.3 billion (December 1994)

Operating units   Has full ownership of one tertiary hospital (903 beds), two acute care community hospitals (534 beds), two specialty hospitals (165 beds), two nursing homes, two skilled nursing facilities, thirteen independent pharmacies, twenty-seven independent laboratories, twenty-seven diagnostic imaging centers, four ambulatory surgery centers, eight IPAs, three PHOs, thirty-six ambulatory care centers offering primary and specialty care, and one of each of the following: home health care agency, durable medical equipment company, PPO, and dialysis company.

Also owns institutes/centers that conduct research on improving the process of health care delivery, including the Center for Health System Studies, Biostatistics, Research Epidemiology, and Medical Informatics (BREMI), the Center for Clinical Effectiveness (CCE), and the new Center for Health Promotion and Disease Prevention (CHPDP).

Managed care Owns Health Alliance Plan (HAP), the largest HMO in Michigan, covering approximately 450,000 of the 950,000 HMO managed care enrollees in the Detroit metropolitan area. In addition, Health Alliance Plan also owns Medical Value Plan (MVP), a nonprofit HMO in Toledo, Ohio, which has 35,000 members.

Mercy Health Services

Headquarters Farmington Hills, Michigan

Area(s) served Michigan, Iowa, Indiana, New York, Illinois, and Nebraska

Total revenues $2.0 billion (June 1994)

Total assets $2.0 billion (June 1994)

Operating units Has majority or full ownership of twenty-three acute care hospitals and one specialty hospital, and manages an additional twelve acute care hospitals and one specialty hospital (total of 5,464 licensed acute care beds in the acute care hospitals owned and operated by MHS). Other units owned and operated by MHS include seventeen nursing homes, fifteen skilled nursing facilities, one home health care agency (Amicare Home Healthcare Company—with several operating units providing home health services; AHHC also provides durable medical equipment services), eleven independent pharmacies, one independent laboratory, twenty-two diagnostic imaging centers, one ambulatory surgery center, twelve physician-hospital organizations and one philanthropic foundation.

Managed care   Owns three managed care plans through its Mercy Alternative subsidiary: Care Choices HMO, developed in 1985 and licensed in 1986; Preferred Choices PPO, developed in 1988; and Preferred Choices Options, a self-insured point-of-service product developed in 1994. As of December 1993, there were 10,906 enrollees in Care Choices HMO in Iowa, 125,282 enrollees in Care Choices HMO in Michigan, and 23,000 enrollees in Preferred Choices PPO. Estimated enrollment for Preferred Choices Options was 3,000–5,000.

Sentara Health System

Headquarters   Norfolk, Virginia

Area(s) served   Hampton Roads area of Virginia

Total revenues $611.4 million (April 1994)

Total assets $753.4 million (April 1994)

Operating units   Has full or majority ownership in four acute care hospitals (with a total of 1,513 licensed acute care beds), six nursing homes, four ambulatory surgery centers, four retirement centers, two single-specialty group practices, two HMOs, and one of each of the following: home health care agency, durable medical equipment company, independent pharmacy, and independent laboratory. Also manages two other single-specialty group practices.

Managed care   Owns Sentara Health Plan, a ten-site primary care staff-model HMO covering 47,000 members; Sentara Mental Health Management, covering over 120,000 capitated lives; Sentara Direct Contracting, which manages and negotiates managed care contracts for Sentara hospitals, covering over 20,000 lives; also has 80 percent ownership in OPTIMA Health Plan, an IPA-model HMO covering over 70,000 members.

Sharp HealthCare

Headquarters   San Diego, California

Area(s) served   Greater San Diego metropolitan area

Total revenues $648.5 million (September 1994)

Total assets $681.9 million (September 1994)

Operating units   Has full ownership of four acute care hospitals (with 1,416 licensed beds), one specialty hospital, four skilled nursing facilities, eighteen medical clinics, eight urgent care centers, two multi-specialty group practices, two single-specialty group practices, one HMO, one home health care agency, one extended care facility, and one hospice. Manages two acute care hospitals. Has minority ownership in a diagnostic imaging center and an ambulatory surgery center. Manages a multispecialty group practice and is affiliated with two single-specialty group practices and two staff-model IPAs. Additional facilities include the Center for Health Promotion, San Diego Regional Cancer Center, Institute for Human Potential and Mind Body Medicine, and the Center for Sports Medicine.

Managed care   Owns and operates its own HMO, Knox-Keene. Also has 325,000 covered lives (capitated) through sixty to seventy managed care contracts.

Special Note   At time of publication, Sharp had signed a letter of intent with Columbia/HCA to implement a 50/50 joint venture ownership of four of Sharp's six hospitals.

Sisters of Providence

Headquarters   Seattle, Washington

Areas served   Alaska, California, Oregon, and Washington, with the majority of its operating units concentrated in the latter two states

Total revenues $1.4 billion (December 1994)

Total assets $1.7 billion (December 1994)

Operating units   Owns fourteen acute care hospitals (3,524 licensed beds), eleven skilled nursing facilities (1,172 long-term beds), nine home health care agencies, two HMOs, two PPOs, two multisite primary care group practices (one in Oregon, one in Washington), two durable medical equipment companies, one retirement center, and one independent laboratory. Manages one skilled nursing facility, one home care agency, and two acute care hospitals.

Managed care   Has 100 percent ownership of the Good Health Plan of Washington (an HMO with 32,000 members); Providence Health Care (a health plan for Medicaid enrollees with 49,505 enrollees); Sound Health (a PPO with 335,000 covered lives); the Good Health Plan of Oregon (an HMO with approximately 108,000 members); and Vantage (Providence Health System's Oregon PPO, with 242,000 members)

Sutter Health

Headquarters   Sacramento, California

Area(s) served   Sacramento, Central Valley, Bay Area, and Northern California regions

Total revenues $1.0 billion (December 1994)

Total assets $1.2 billion (December 1994)

Operating units   Has majority or full ownership in twelve acute care hospitals (total of 1,524 licensed beds), two psychiatric hospitals (total of 226 beds), four skilled nursing facilities, one adult day care center, one home health care agency, one retirement center, five philanthropic foundations, three biomedical engineering centers, two community clinics, one durable medical equipment company, five medical foundations (which include eight multispecialty medical groups), and three diagnostic imaging centers. Has a joint venture interest in an outpatient surgery center with locations in four states. Has partial ownership of a clinical laboratory company.

Managed care Owns 100 percent of Sutter Preferred Insurance Administrators (third-party administrators with 23,726 covered lives), 100 percent of Sutter Preferred Health and Life (an insurance company with 30,389 covered lives), and 75 percent of Sutter Preferred/OMNI (an HMO with a total of 106,362 covered lives). Sutter Health has 252,000 covered lives under capitation contracts through partially owned and non-owned products.

UniHealth

Headquarters Burbank, California

Area(s) served Five-county region of Southern California (recently entered the Northern California market with the intent to establish a statewide physician delivery system)

Total revenues $1.4 billion (FY 1994)

Total assets $1.6 billion (FY 1994)

Operating units Owns nine acute care hospitals (total of 2,662 licensed beds), CliniShare (a home health and disease management company), and ElderMed America (provides consulting services for the senior market). Affiliated with seven medical groups or IPAs, representing over 2,300 physicians, including nearly 1,000 primary care physicians.

Managed care Has full ownership of CareAmerica Health Plans, Inc., with approximately 235,000 enrollees. Has a significant interest in PacifiCare Health Systems, Inc., a publicly owned HMO with more than 1.5 million members as of March 1995. Has contracts with many third-party payers and managed care plans in an effort to establish long-term strategic partnerships with the payer community.

Resource B

• •

Collecting the Data

Note: The self-administered questionnaires and original data collection instruments as well as more information regarding the concepts and measures used in the study are available at cost by contacting: the Health Systems Integration Project, Attn.: Robin Gillies, Ph.D., Health Services Management, Kellogg Graduate School of Management, Leverone Hall, Northwestern University, 2001 Sheridan Road, Evanston, IL 60208–2007.

Data Collection Source	Type	Date	Content or Concepts Measured
Background information questionnaire	Open-ended questionnaire completed by each system; used to compile system profile	12/90	History and vision
			Success factors
			Major obstacles
			Study interests
			System information—when system formed; number of operating units by type; number of beds; operating revenues
Background profile material from each system	System and operating unit strategic plans, annual reports, consolidated audited financial statements, system internal communication instruments, operating-unit internal communication instruments, corporate organization chart, management organization chart, etc. Archival, content analysis	12/90 12/91 12/92 12/93	System strategic plan
			Operating-unit strategic plans
			Annual reports
			Consolidated audited financial statements
			System internal communication instruments
			Operating-unit internal communication instruments
			Corporate organization chart
			Management organization chart

Strategy measures questionnaire	Self-administered structured questionnaire (given to corporate management, noncorporate management, key board members, key physicians—system and operating units)	4/91–10/91 1/94–4/94	Strategy (1991) Strategic orientation (1991; 1994) Differentiation, low cost (1991)
Perceived systemness and integration measures questionnaire	Self-administered structured questionnaire (given to corporate management, noncorporate management, key board members [primarily 1991], key physicians—system and operating units)	4/91–10/91 7/92–9/92 1/94–4/94	Perceived system integration (1991 and 1992—culture, financial management resource allocation, financial management operating policies, human resource, information systems, marketing, quality improvement, strategic planning, support services; overall functional, physician-system, and clinical; 1994—quality assurance, information systems, physician-system integration, and clinical integration items only) Perceived effectiveness (1991) Systemness (1991)

Data Collection Source (*Cont.*)	Type	Date	Content or Concepts Measured
System office–unit relationship measures questionnaire	Self-administered structured questionnaire (given to corporate management, noncorporate management, key board members [primarily 1991], key physicians—system and operating units)	4/91–10/91	Centralization
Site visit interviews	Interviews (corporate management, noncorporate management, key board members, key physicians—system and operating units)	6/91–10/91	System culture Clinical integration Perceived systemness integration Managed care Centralization
Managed care questionnaires	Interview (key managed care interviewees during site visit)	6/91–10/91	Managed care—provide more specific rank ordering of attributes most desired by purchasers, etc.
System VP-Strategy questionnaire	HealthOne questionnaire (system VP Strategy—collected at site visit interview)	6/91–10/91	Standardization of services and activities across the system

Historical evolution of System I and II	Table completed by system VP-Strategy	6/91–10/91 1/92	Acquisitions and mergers versus internal development; divestitures
Objective performance and related measures	Tables completed by key people at each system or operating unit	4/92–9/92 7/93–10/93	Culture Managed care Physician-system integration Examples: economic involvement, including physician utilization activity, joint venture activity, physician benefits, shared contracts; administrative involvement; group practice formation; shared accountability Clinical integration Examples: clinical protocol development; medical records uniformity and accessibility; clinical outcomes data collection and utilization; clinical programming and planning efforts; shared clinical support services; shared clinical service lines

Data Collection Source (*Cont.*)	Type	Date	Content or Concepts Measured
Consolidated balance sheets	Financial information from balance sheets for system and selected operating units provided by system VP-Strategy	FY 1991 FY 1992	Financial performance measures Cost/case, total revenue, productivity, cash flow/net, cash flow/total, debt coverage, liquidity, leverage, total margin, charge/day
Financial supplemental information	Table completed by system VP-Strategy	FY 1991 FY 1992	System and operating-unit patient volume and productivity measures
Market competitiveness and contextual variables questionnaire	Tables completed by each system providing information, plus data drawn from the American Hospital Association Guide (1992), MGMA 1992 directory, AGPA 1992 directory, AMA Physician Characteristics and Distribution in the United States (1992), and the Interstudy Competitive Edge (1992); data compiled in Market Competitiveness and Contextual Variables sourcebook	1/93	System evolution Average length of time of units with system Top management team stability Geographic concentration of units Market environment System governance Strategy

Barriers survey	6/93	Survey completed by system executives and operating-unit executives/manager	Eight barriers and thirty exhibited behaviors assessed as to degree to which each is a problem within system
Organizational culture questionnaire	1/94–4/94	Self-administered structured questionnaire (given to corporate management, noncorporate management, key physicians—system and operating units)	Organizational culture types: Group Developmental Rational Hierarchical
Clinical integration site visit interviews	5/94–7/94	Interviews—system CEO; hospital COO; system and hospital VPs for clinical affairs; system and hospital VPs for quality assurance; system and hospital VPs for information technology; hospital-level physicians, nurses, and support personnel for five clinical service lines; head of physician group; representative of home health; head of system insurance plan)	Clinical integration, including: Population health status needs CQI/TQM Physician involvement Clinical information systems Technology assessment Management and governance support Case management/coordinated care management

Data Collection Source (Cont.)	Type	Date	Content or Concepts Measured
			Guideline/protocol development and clinical reengineering
			Performance/outcome measurement
			Organization of service line
			Best practices

Resource C

• •

Some Related Readings

From the Health Systems Integration Study

Devers, K. J., and others. "Implementing Organized Delivery Systems: An Integration Scorecard." *Health Care Management Review*, 1994, *19*(3), 7–20.

Gillies, R. R., and others. "Conceptualizing and Measuring Integration: Findings from the Health Systems Integration Study." *Hospital & Health Services Administration*, 1993, *38*(4), 467–489.

Shortell, S. M., Gillies, R. R., and Anderson, D. A. "The New World of Managed Care: Creating Organized Delivery Systems." *Health Affairs*, 1994, *13*(5), 46–64.

Shortell, S. M., Gillies, R. R., and Devers, K. J. "Reinventing the American Hospital." *The Milbank Quarterly*, 1995, *73*(2), 131–160.

Shortell, S. M., and others. "The Holographic Organization." *Healthcare Forum Journal*, 1993, *36*(2), 20–26.

Shortell, S. M., and others. "Creating Organized Delivery Systems: The Barriers and Facilitators." *Hospital & Health Services Administration*, 1993, *38*(4), 447–466.

Related Works

Coddington, D. C., Moore, K. D., and Fischer, E. A. *Integrated Health Care: Reorganizing the Physician, Hospital and Health Plan Relationship.* Englewood, CO: Center for Research in Ambulatory Health Care Administration, 1994.

Kaluzny, A. D., Zuckerman, H. S., and Ricketts, T. C., III (eds.). *Partners for the Dance: Forming Strategic Alliances in Health Care*. Ann Arbor, MI: Health Administration Press, 1995.

Moscovice, I., Christianson, J., Johnson, J., Kralewski, J., and Manning, W. *Building Rural Hospital Networks*. Ann Arbor, MI: Health Administration Press, 1995.

References

Abraham, L. K. *Mama Might Be Better Off Dead*. Chicago: University of Chicago Press, 1994.

Advisory Board Company. *The Grand Alliance: Vertical Integration Strategies for Physicians and Health Systems*. Washington, D.C.: Advisory Board Company, 1993.

Alexander, J. A., Burns, L. R., and Zuckerman, H. S. *Phase One—Survey Results*. Working Paper Series, no. 7. Network for Health Care Management, Arizona State University, 1995.

Alexander, J. A., and others. *Phase One Summary Report of Physicians Survey*. Network on Health Management Education, Center for Health Management Research, Arizona State University, 1995.

Allen, D., and Weber, D. "Twin Cities Hospital Breaks Down Ambulatory Care, Overcomes Fears of Outpatient Care." *Health Care System Strategy Report*, Jan. 6, 1995, pp. 1–4.

Alpha Center. "Washington State 70 Point Ambitious Public Health Improvement Plan." *State Initiatives*. Washington, D.C.: Alpha Center, Jan./Feb. 1995, pp. 8–9.

American Hospital Association. "Assessing Health Status: A Five Phase Model." *Hospitals & Health Networks*, Dec. 20, 1993a, 67(24), 29.

American Hospital Association. *Transforming Health Care Delivery: Toward Community Care Networks.* Chicago: American Hospital Association, 1993b.

American Practice Management (APM). *Health System Market Profile Characteristics.* New York: APM, 1993.

Argote, L. "Group and Organizational Learning Curves: Individual, System and Environmental Components." *British Journal of Social Psychology*, 1993, *32*, 31–51.

Argyris, C. *Reasoning, Learning, and Action: Individual and Organizational.* San Francisco: Jossey-Bass, 1982.

Bader, B. "Population-Based Health Improvement: Group Health Cooperative's Eight-Step Process." *The Quality Letter*, December 1994–January 1995, 13.

Bader, B. S., and Associates. "Measuring and Improving Community Health." *The Quality Letter for Healthcare Leaders*, June 1994, 6(5), 1–40.

Barney, J. "Strategic Factor Markets: Expectation, Luck, and Business Strategies." *Management Science*, 1986, *32*, 1231–1241.

Bartling, A. C. "Integrated Delivery Systems: Fact or Fiction." *Healthcare Executive*, May/June 1995, pp. 6–11.

Barsness, Z. I., Shortell, S. M., Gillies, R. R., and others. "The Quality March—National Survey Profiles Quality Improvement Activities." *Hospitals & Health Networks*, Dec. 1993, pp. 52–55.

Begun, J. W., and Lippincott, R. C. *Strategic Adaptation in the Health Professions: Meeting the Challenges of Change.* San Francisco: Jossey-Bass, 1993.

Bethell, C. A. *Typology and Discussion of Community Health Initiatives: The New Challenge for Public Health Agencies and Health Systems.* Unpublished working paper, University of Chicago, 1995.

Bettis, R. A., and Prahalad, C. K. "The Dominant Logic: Retrospective and Extension." *Strategic Management Journal*, 1995, *16*, 5–14.

Blumenthal, D., and Scheck, A. C. *Improving Clinical Practice: Total Quality Management and the Physician.* San Francisco: Jossey-Bass, 1995.

Blumstein, J. F. "Health Care Reform and Competing Visions of Medical Care: Antitrust and State Provider Cooperative Legislation." *Cornell Law Review,* 1994, 9(6), 1459–1506.

Bradford, D. L., and Cohen, A. R. *Managing for Excellence.* New York: Wiley, 1984.

Bray, N., and others. "An Examination of Winners and Losers Under Medicare Prospective Payment System." *Health Care Management Review,* 1994, *19*(3), 7–20.

Brown, L. "Integration for What? Public Policy Meets Integrated Service Networks." Paper presented at Robert Wood Johnson Foundation Conference, Washington, D.C., 1994.

Burns, L. R., and Wholey, D. "Matrix Management in Hospitals: Testing Theories of Matrix Structure and Development." *Administrative Science Quarterly,* 1989, *34,* 349–368.

Byrne, J. A. "The Horizontal Corporation." *Business Week,* Dec. 20, 1993, pp. 76–81.

Cochrane, J. D. "Can Academic Medical Centers Survive?" *Integrated Health Care Report,* Feb. 1995, pp. 1–9.

Cave, D. C. "Vertical Integration Models to Prepare Health Systems for Capitation." *Health Care Management Review,* 1995, *20*(1), 26–39.

Cerne, F. "Engineering a System Culture: Functioning as a System Cultivates Integration." *Hospitals & Health Networks,* 1994, 68(6), 36–39.

Charns, M. P., and Smith-Tewsbury, L. J. *Collaborative Management in Healthcare: Implementing the Integrative Organization.* San Francisco: Jossey-Bass, 1993.

Coddington, D. C., Moore, K. D., and Fischer, E. A. *Integrated Health Care: Reorganizing the Physician, Hospital, Health Plan Relationship.* Englewood, Colo.: Center for Research in Ambulatory Health Care Administration (CRACHA), MGMA, 1994.

Coile, R. C. "The Five Stages of Managed Care: Organizing for Capitation and Health Reform." *Hospital Strategy Report,* Sept. 1994, 6, 1–8.

Coile, R. C. "Age Wave: Organizing Integrated Care Networks for an Aging Society." *Health Trends*, 1995, *7*(6), 1–8.

Committee on the Costs of Medical Care. *Medical Care for the American People: The Final Report of the Committee on the Costs of Medical Care.* Publication no. 18. Chicago: University of Chicago Press and the Commission on Medical Education, 1932.

Conrad, D. A. "Coordinating Patient Care Services in Regional Health Systems: The Challenge of Clinical Integration." *Hospital & Health Services Administration*, 1993, *38*(4), 491–508.

Conrad, D. A., and Dowling, W. L. "Vertical Integration in Health Services: Theory and Managerial Implication." *Health Care Management Review*, 1990, *15*, 9–22.

Davis, S. M. *Future Perfect.* Reading, Mass: Addison-Wesley, 1987.

Devers, K. J., and others. "Implementing Organized Delivery Systems: An Integration Scorecard." *Health Care Management Review*, 1994, *19*(3), 7–20.

Dorenfest, S. I. Sheldon I. Dorenfest and Associates, Ltd. *H.C.I.S. Market Review*, 1995.

Drake, D. F. *Reforming the Health Care System: An Interpretive Economic History.* Washington, D.C.: Georgetown University Press, 1994.

Drucker, P. "The Theory of the Business." *Harvard Business Review*, Sept./Oct. 1994, pp. 95–104.

Dukerich, J. M., Golden, B. R., and Shortell, S. M. "The Antecedents and Consequences of Organizational Identification in Vertically Integrated Health Delivery Systems." Working paper presented at the meeting of the Academy of Management, Vancouver, B.C., Canada, Aug. 1995.

Dunham, N. C., Kindig, D. A., and Schulz, R. "The Value of the Physician Executive Role to Organizational Effectiveness and Performance." *Health Care Management Review*, 1994, *19*(4), 56–63.

Ellwood, P. N. "Shattuck Lecture—Outcomes Management: A Technology of Patient Experience." *The New England Journal of Medicine*, 1988, *318*, 1549–1556.

Entin, F. J. Testimony before the Senate Judiciary Sub-Committee on Anti-Trust, Monopolies, and Business Rights, Washington, D.C., Mar. 23, 1994.

Enthoven, A. C. "The History and Principles of Managed Competition." *Health Affairs*, Supplement, 1993, pp. 24–48.

Felsenthal, E. "New Rules Let Hospitals Start Joint Ventures." *Wall Street Journal*, May 14, 1993, p. 31.

Fickenscher, K., and Lagerwey-Voorman, M. "An Overview of Rural Health Care." In S. M. Shortell and U. E. Reinhardt (eds.), *Improving Health Policy and Management: Nine Critical Research Issues for the 1990s*. Ann Arbor, Mich.: Health Administration Press, 1992, pp. 111–150.

Fox, P. D., and Wasserman, J. "Academic Medical Centers and Managed Care: Uneasy Partners." *Health Affairs*, Spring 1993, pp. 85–93.

Fox, W. "Vertical Integration Strategies: More Promising Than Diversification." *Health Care Management Review*, Summer 1989, *14*, 49–56.

Franciscan Health System. *Franciscan Health System Annual Report: Fiscal Year 1994*. Aston, Penn.: Franciscan Health System, 1994.

Freidson, E. *Professional Dominance: The Social Structure of Medical Care*. New York: Atherton Press, 1970a.

Freidson, E. *Profession of Medicine*. New York: HarperCollins, 1970b.

"The Future of Medicine: Peering into 2010." *The Economist*, Mar. 19, 1994, pp. 15–16.

Gardner, K. "A System That 'Walks the Talk.'" Interview with John C. McMeekin and Richard W. Billings. *Trustee*, Apr. 1994, pp. 6–9.

Gillies, R. R., and others. "Conceptualizing and Measuring Integration: Findings from the Health Systems Integration Study." *Hospital & Health Services Administration,* 1993, *38*(4), 467–489.

Goldsmith, J. C. "The Elusive Logic of Integration." *Health Forum Journal,* 1994, *37*(5), 26–31.

Griffith, J. R. "The Infrastructure of Integrated Delivery Systems," *Healthcare Executive,* May/June 1995, pp. 12–17.

Griffith, J. R., Sahney, V. K., and Mohr, R. A. *Reengineering Health Care: Building on CQI.* Ann Arbor, Mich.: Health Administration Press, 1995.

Hall, G., Rosenthal, J., and Wade, J. "How to Make Reengineering Really Work." *Harvard Business Review,* Nov./Dec. 1993, pp. 119–131.

Hambrick, D. C., and Cannella, A. A., Jr. "Strategy Implementation as Substance and Selling." *The Academy of Management Executive,* 1989, *3*(4), 278–285.

Hammer, M., and Champy, J. *Reengineering the Corporation: A Manifesto for Business Revolution.* New York: HarperCollins, 1993.

Handy, C. *The Age of Unreason.* Boston: Harvard Business School Press, 1989.

Hart, G. W., quoted in Iglehart, J. K. "Rapid Changes for Academic Medical Centers." *The New England Journal of Medicine,* 1995, *332*(6), 409.

Healthcare Forum. *What Creates Health? Individuals in Communities Respond.* A national study conducted by Dyg, Inc., for the Healthcare Forum. San Francisco: Healthcare Forum, 1993.

Henry Ford Health System. *Cost-Effectiveness of Integrated Group Practice: A Case Study.* Detroit, Mich.: Henry Ford Medical Group, 1993, p. 7.

Henry Ford Health System. *Henry Ford Health System 1994 System Report.* Detroit, Mich.: Henry Ford Health System, 1994, pp. 6, 8.

Henry Ford Health System. *Henry Ford Balanced Scorecard Measures.* 1995.

Hing, E. *Characteristics of Elderly Home Health Patients: Preliminary Data from the 1992 National Home and Hospice Survey.* Hyattsville, Md.: National Center for Health Statistics, U.S. Department of Health and Human Services, 1994.

Hofstede, G. *Cultures and Organizations.* New York: McGraw-Hill, 1991.

Hospital Association of Pennsylvania. *A Guide for Assessing and Improving Health Status.* Harrisburg, Penn.: Policy Research Department, Hospital Association of Pennsylvania, 1993.

Hospital Research and Educational Trust (HRET). *Community Action Learning Laboratories.* Chicago: American Hospital Association, 1994.

"Hospitals, Integrated Delivery Systems, and Their Evolving Role in Health Plans: Braving the World of Insurance Regulation." Washington, D.C.: Policy Development Group, American Hospital Association, 1995, p. 36.

Integrated Health Care Report. "How Can Hospitals Survive?" *Integrated Health Care Report,* July 1994, p. 2.

Huber, G. P., and Glick, W. H. *Organizational Change and Redesign: Ideas and Insights for Improving Performance.* New York: Oxford University Press, 1993.

Hughes, E.F.X. *New Leadership in Health Care Management: The Physician Executives II.* Tampa, Fla.: American College of Physician Executives, 1994.

Hurley, R. E. "Towards a Seamless Health Care Delivery System." *Frontiers of Health Services Management.* Summer 1993, pp. 5–35.

Iezzoni, L. I. *Risk Adjustment for Measuring Health Care Outcomes.* Ann Arbor, MI: Health Administration Press, 1994.

Iglehart, J. K. "The American Health Care System: Community Hospitals." *The New England Journal of Medicine,* 1993, *329*(5), 372–376.

Iglehart, J. K. "Rapid Changes for Academic Medical Centers." *The New England Journal of Medicine,* 1995, *332*(6), 407–411.

Institute for Alternative Futures. *Healthy People in a Healthy World: The Belmont Vision for Health Care in America*. Alexandria, Va.: Institute for Alternative Futures, 1992.

Institute for Health Care Quality Improvement. Community Healthcare Collaborative, Boston, Mass., 1994.

Institute for the Future. *Health Care Outcomes, Year Seven: First Theme Report*. Menlo Park, Calif.: Institute for the Future, 1993a, p. 28.

Institute for the Future. "Integrated Medical Systems: The Next Generation of Managed Care." Unpublished report, Menlo Park, Calif., 1993b.

Institute of Medicine. *Prenatal Care: Reaching Mothers, Reaching Infants*. Washington, D.C.: National Academy Press, 1988, p. 232.

Institute of Medicine. *Healthy People 2000: Citizens Chart the Course*. Ed. M. A. Stoto, R. Behrens, and C. Rosemont. Washington, D.C.: National Academy Press, 1990.

Jewish Healthcare Foundation. "Health Environmental Scan." *Jewish Healthcare Foundation*. Pittsburgh, Penn., 1995, pp. 23, 25.

Johnson & Johnson. *Redefining the Health Care System*. New Brunswick, N.J.: Johnson & Johnson, 1994.

Jones, W. J., and Mayerhofer, J. J. *Guide to Population-Based Planning, Part I*. San Francisco: New Century Healthcare Institute, April 10, 1994.

Jones, W. J., and Mayerhofer, J. J. "Regional Health Care Systems: Implications for Health Care Reform." *Managed Care Quarterly*, 1994, 2(1), 31–44.

Kaluzny, A. D., Zuckerman, H. S., and Ricketts, T. C., III (eds.). *Partners for the Dance: Forming Strategic Alliances in Health Care*. Ann Arbor, Mich.: Health Administration Press, 1995.

Kaluzny, A. D., and others. *Improving Community Cancer Care: Managing a Strategic Alliance*. San Francisco: Jossey-Bass, 1996.

Kane, V. L. "An Older America: Strategic Challenges for the Acute Care Hospital." *Health Management Quarterly*, Winter 1994, pp. 9–12. Deerfield, Ill.: Baxter Foundation.

Kane, V. L., and others. *The Role of the Hospital in an Aging Society*. Report prepared by Age Wave, Emeryville, Calif. Deerfield, Ill.: Baxter Foundation, 1994.

Kanter, R. M. "Becoming Pals: Pooling, Aligning, and Linking Across Companies." *Academy of Management Executive*, Aug. 1989, 3, 183–193.

Kaplan, R. S., and Norton, D. P. "The Balanced Scorecard: Measures that Drive Performance." *Harvard Business Review*, Jan./Feb. 1992, pp. 71–79.

Kaplan, R. S., and Norton, D. P. "Putting the Balanced Scorecard to Work." *Harvard Business Review*, Sept./Oct. 1993, pp. 134–137.

Kennedy, M. "Reengineering in Health Care." *The Quality Letter*, 1994, 6(7), 2–10.

Kofman, F., and Senge, P. M. "Communities of Commitment: The Heart of Learning Organizations." *Organizational Dynamics*, 1993, 22(2), 5–23.

Kotha, S. "Mass Customization: Implementing the Emerging Paradigm for Competitive Advantage." *Strategic Management Journal*, Summer 1995, 16, 21–42.

Kralewski, J., and Wingert, T. D. "Some Preliminary Observations Regarding the Impact of Managed Care and Provider Consolidation on the Minneapolis/St. Paul, Minnesota Health Care System." Working draft, Institute for Health Services Research, University of Minnesota, May 1995.

Kralovec, J. "The Critical Role Information Systems Play in Reengineering Efforts." *The Quality Letter*, 1994, 6(7), 11–13.

Lathrop, P. *Restructuring Health Care: A Patient-Focused Paradigm*. San Francisco: Jossey-Bass, 1993.

Leape, L. L. "Error in Medication." *Journal of the American Medical Association*, Dec. 23, 1994, 274, 1851.

Leatt, P., Pink, G. H., and Naylor, C. D. *Integrated Delivery Systems—Has Their Time Come in Canada?* Technical Report No. 95–01. Toronto: Hospital Management Research Unit, Department of Health Administration, University of Toronto, June 1995, pp. 1–14.

Luke, R. D. "The Emergence of Integrated Health Systems." Presentation to MDI Emerging Medical Technologies Program, Mar. 18, 1994.

Lumsdon, K. "Crash Course: Piecing Together the Continuum of Care." *Hospitals & Health Networks*, Nov. 20, 1994, pp. 26–28.

Lumsdon, K. "Hard Labor." *Hospitals & Health Networks*. Apr. 5, 1995, pp. 34–42.

McKnight, J. "Two Tools for Well-Being: Health Systems and Communities." Paper presented at the Conference on Medicine for the 21st Century, American Medical Association, Annenberg Washington Program, U.S. Environmental Protection Agency, and W. K. Kellogg Foundation, Feb. 6, 1992.

McNerney, W. J. "Community Health Initiatives Are Widespread, Challenging Our Sense of Civic Obligation." *Frontiers of Health Services Management*, Summer 1995, pp. 39–44.

Mercy Health Services. *Mercy Health Services Strategic/Financial Play.* FY 1996–FY 1998, 1995, p. 6.

Miles, R. E., and Snow, C. C. *Organizational Strategy, Structure, and Processes.* New York: McGraw-Hill, 1978.

Miles, R. E., and Snow, C. C. "Network Organizations: New Concepts for New Forms." *California Management Review*, 1986, Spring, pp. 62–73.

Miles, R. E., and Snow, C. C. *Fit, Failure, and the Hall of Fame: How Companies Succeed or Fail.* New York: Free Press, 1994.

Molinari, C., Alexander, J., Morlock, L., and Lyles, C. A. "Does the Hospital Board Need a Doctor? The Influence of Physician Board Participation on Hospital Financial Performance." *Medical Care*, 1995, 33(2), 170–185.

Mor, V., and Rice, C. "Physician Use Among Patients Receiving Cancer Chemotherapy." *Cancer*, 1993, 71(1), 219–225.

Morgan, G. *Images of Organization*. Beverly Hills, Calif.: Sage Library of Social Research, 1986.

Morlock, L., and Alexander, J. "Models of Governance in Multihospital System." *Medical Care*, 1986, 24(12), 1118–1135.

Moscovice, I. *Integrated Health Services Delivery and Financing Approaches in Rural Environments*. Report commissioned by the National Institute for Health Care Management, Washington, D.C., June 1994.

Moscovice, I., and others. *Building Rural Hospital Networks*. Ann Arbor, Mich.: Health Administration Press, 1995.

National Civic League. Ten Guiding Principles Created by the Alliance for National Renewal Partners Initiative, Denver, 1995.

Nelson, E. C., and others. "Report Cards or Instrument Panels: Who Needs What?" *Jt Comm J Qual Improv*, 1995, 21(4), 155–166.

"1994 Cal ALS 812; 1994 Cal SB 697; Stats 1994 Ch 812." *Deerings, California Code Annotated*. Advance Legislative Service, Bancroft-Whitney Company, 1994.

"New Governance Structure Announced to Guide Sentara and Hampton Roads into a New Era of Health Care." *Network Special Edition*. Norfolk, VA: Sentara Health System, July 25, 1994.

O'Brien, J. L., Shortell, S. M., and Hughes, E.F.X. "An Evaluation of New England Medical Center's Patient Care Restructuring Project." Final report by the Center for Health Services and Policy Research and the J. L. Kellogg Graduate School of Management, Northwestern University. Submitted to the Pew Charitable Trusts, Philadelphia, Penn., May 2, 1994.

O'Brien, J. L., Shortell, S. M., and others. "An Integrative Model for Organization-Wide Quality Improvement: Lessons from the Field." *Quality Management in Health Care*, 1995, 3(4), 19–30.

Office of Technology Assessment, U.S. Congress. *Identifying Health Technologies That Work: Searching for Evidence*. OTA-H-608. Washington, D.C.: U.S. Government Printing Office, 1991.

O'Hare, W. P. "America's Minorities—The Demographics of Diversity." *Population Bulletin*, 1992, 47(4), 1–46.

O'Neil, E. "Health Professions Education for the Future: Schools in Service to the Nation." Center for the Health Professions, University of California, San Francisco: Pew Health Professions Commissions, February 1993.

Padden, M. D. "A Focus on Antitrust, Legal Perspectives in Provider Networks." Unpublished paper, Center for Health Administration Studies, University of Chicago, Winter 1995 workshops.

Parsons, M. L. "Arizona's UMC Model of Patient-Centered Care Thrives After Four Years." *Strategies For Health Care Excellence*, Apr. 1995, pp. 1–8.

Peck, M. S. *The Different Drum: Community-Making and Peace.* New York: Simon & Schuster, 1987.

Pointer, D. D., Alexander, J. A., and Zuckerman, H. S. "Loosening the Gordian Knot of Governance in Integrated Health Care Delivery Systems." *Frontiers of Health Services Management*, 1995, 11(3), pp. 3–37.

Prahalad, C. K., and Bettis, R. A. "The Dominant Logic: A New Linkage Between Diversity and Performance." *Strategic Management Journal*, 1986, 7, 485–501.

"President's Message." *Sutter Health Annual Report.* Sacramento, Calif.: Sutter Health, 1992.

"Progressive Portland." *Modern Healthcare*, June 19, 1995, p. 118.

Prahalad, C. K., and Hamel, G. "The Core Competence of the Corporation." *Harvard Business Review*, May–June 1990, pp. 79–91.

Quinn, R. E., and Kimberly, J. R. "Paradox, Planning, and Perseverance: Guidelines for Managerial Practices." In J. R. Kimberly amd R. E. Quinn (eds.), *Managing Organization Transitions.* Homewood, Ill.: Dow Jones-Irwin, 1984, pp. 295–313.

Reinertsen, J. L. "Living Guidelines." *Healthcare Forum Journal*, Nov./Dec. 1994, pp. 58–59.

Risk, R. R., and Francis, C. P. "Transforming a Hospital Facility Company into an Integrated Medical Care Organization." *Managed Care Quarterly,* 1994, *2*(4), 12–23.

Rundall, T. G., and Schauffler, H. H. "Incorporating Health Promotion and Disease Prevention into Integrated Delivery Systems." Unpublished report presented to the Center for Health Management Research, Tempe, Ariz., June 1995.

"Running the Integrated Delivery System Gauntlet." *Medical Staff Strategy Report,* 1994, *3*(2), 3.

Scheffler, R., and Waitzkin, N. *The Health Workforce.* Berkeley: University of California Press, 1996.

Schultz, D., Napiewocki, L., and Nerenz, D. "Measuring Physician Integration in Health Care Systems." Paper presented at the annual meeting of the Association for Health Services Research, Washington, D.C., June 14, 1994.

Scott, L. "Duplication Hard to Limit Despite Hospital Mergers." *Modern Health Care,* Mar. 13, 1995, pp. 42–43.

Scott, W. R. "Managing Professional Work: Three Models of Control for Healthcare Organizations." *Health Services Research,* 1982, *17*(3), 213–240.

Senge, P. *The Fifth Discipline.* New York: Doubleday/Currency, 1990.

Shalowitz, J. I. Presentations for Executive Education Program, Allen Center, Northwestern University, 1993.

Shalowitz, J. I. Presentations for Executive Education Program, Allen Center, Northwestern University, 1994.

Sherman, V. C. *Creating the New American Hospital: A Time for Greatness.* San Francisco: Jossey-Bass, 1993.

Shortell, S. M. "The Evolution of Hospital Systems: Unfulfilled Promises and Self-Fulfilling Prophecies." *Medical Care Review,* 1988, *45*(2), 177–214.

Shortell, S. M. *Effective Hospital-Physician Relationships.* Ann Arbor, Mich.: Health Administration Press, 1991.

Shortell, S. M., Gillies, R. R., and Anderson, D. A. "The New World of Managed Care: Creating Organized Delivery Systems." *Health Affairs*, 1994, *13*(5), 46–64.

Shortell, S. M., Gillies, R. R., and Devers, K. J. "Reinventing the American Hospital." *The Milbank Quarterly*, 1995, *73*(2), 131–160.

Shortell, S. M., Anderson, D. A., and others. "The Holographic Organization." *Healthcare Forum Journal*, Mar./Apr. 1993, pp. 20–26.

Shortell, S. M., Gillies, R. R., and others. "Creating Organized Delivery Systems: The Barriers and Facilitators." *Hospital & Health Services Administration*, 1993, *38*(4), 447–466.

Shortell, S. M., Levin, D. Z., O'Brien, J. L., and Hughes, E. F. X. "Assessing the Evidence on CQI: Is the Glass Half Empty or Half Full?" *Hospital & Health Services Administration*, Spring 1995, *40*(1), 4–24.

Shortell, S. M., Morrison, E. M., and Friedman, B. *Strategic Choices for America's Hospitals: Managing Change in Turbulent Times*. San Francisco: Jossey-Bass, 1990.

Shortell, S. M., O'Brien, J. L., and others. "Assessing the Impact of Continuous Quality Improvement/Total Quality Management: Concept Versus Implementation." *Health Services Research*, 1995a, *30*(2), 377–401.

Shortell, S. M., and others. "Physician Involvement in Quality Improvement: Issues, Challenges, and Recommendations." In D. Blumenthal and A. C. Scheck (eds.), *Improving Clinical Practice: Total Quality Management and the Physician*. San Francisco: Jossey-Bass, 1995b, pp. 205–228.

Sigmond, R. "Back to the Future: Partnerships and Coordination for Community Health Benefit." *Frontiers of Health Services Management*, Summer 1995, pp. 5–36.

Simons, R. *Levers of Control, How Managers Use Innovative Control Systems to Drive Strategic Renewal*. Boston: Harvard Business School Press, 1995.

Smith, C. S. "The Impact of an Ambulatory Firm's System on Quality and Continuity of Care." *Medical Care*, 1995, *33*(3), 221–226.

Smith-Daniels, V., Schweikhart, S., and Kronenfeld, J. *Restructuring Patient Care Delivery*. Report to the Center for Health Management Research, Arizona State University, and the Network for Health Management Education, Aug. 31, 1994.

Southwick, K. "Case Study: Putting the Pieces in Place for Regional Integration." *Strategies for Healthcare Excellence*, 1994, 7(1), 1–7.

Stalk, G., Evans, P., and Shulman, L. "Competing on Capabilities: The New Rules of Corporate Strategy." *Harvard Business Review*, Mar./Apr. 1992, pp. 57–69.

Starr, P. *The Social Transformation of American Medicine*. New York: Basic Books, 1983.

Stevens, R. *American Medicine and the Public Interest*. New Haven, Conn.: Yale University Press, 1971.

Thompson, J. D. *Organizations in Action*. New York: McGraw-Hill, 1967.

U.S. General Accounting Office. *Antitrust in the Health Care Industry*. Washington, D.C.: U.S. General Accounting Office, 1995.

Voluntary Hospitals of America. *Integration: Market Forces and Critical Success Factors*. Irving, Tex.: Voluntary Hospitals of America, 1994, pp. 1–6.

Ware, J. E. *SR–36 Health Survey, Manual & Interpretation Guide*. Boston: Nimrod, 1993.

Washington State Health Care Commission. *Final report to Booth Gardner and the Washington State Legislature*. Olympia, Wash.: Washington State Health Care Commission, Nov. 30, 1992, p. 86.

Weber, D. O., and Weber, A. L. "Compendium of Patient Focused Care Demonstrations." *Health Care Forum*, Sept./Oct. 1994, pp. 47–61.

Webster's Ninth New Collegiate Dictionary. Springfield, Mass.: Merriam-Webster, 1990.

Wegner, D. M. "Transactive Memory: A Contemporary Analysis of the Group Mind." In B. Mullen and G.R. Goethals (eds.), *Theories of Group Behavior*. Hillsdale, N.J.: Erlbaum, 1986, pp. 185–208.

Weil, T. P. "Close to a Bull's Eye—A Concurring Opinion." *Health Care Management Review*, Spring 1995, 20(2), 35–44.

Williams, J. B. "Guidelines for Managing Integration." *Health Care Forum Journal*, Mar./Apr. 1992, pp. 39–47.

Williamson, J. "Medical Quality Management Systems in Perspective." In J. B. Couch (ed.), *Health Care Quality Management for the 21st Century*. Tampa, Fla.: American College of Physician Executives, 1991, pp. 23–72.

Zelman, W. "Private Markets: Public Issues." Working paper, Agency for Health Care Policy and Research, Rockville, Md., 1995.

Index

operating-unit commitment to, 65–66, 70–71, 81; participants' perspectives on, 61; performance assessment of, 75; and personnel training, 67, 75; primary findings regarding, 59–61; purpose of, 57–58; and standardization, 62–63; and strategic orientation, 50; strategic planning for, 68–69, 77; in study organizations, described, 75–91; success factors in, 68–75, 79–80, 83–84, 88–91; and system culture, 49–50, 71–72, 77, 81–82, 88–89; understanding of, lack of, 64. *See also* Integration
"Future of Medicine, The: Peering into 2010," 282, 283–285

G

Galilean Shift, 28
Gardner, K., 21
General Electric, 45
Geographic concentration: and clinical integration, 54, 156, 162, 166, 181–182; and functional integration, 51, 66–67; and physician-system integration, 51–52, 99
Gillies, R. R., 7, 22, 30, 51, 56, 61, 95, 99, 102, 106, 128, 163, 234, 237, 296, 335
Glick, W. H., 185
Golden, B. R., 115
Goldsmith, J. C., 7, 232
Governance structures: alignment of, with system, 23, 228, 277–278; challenges of, 233–242, 277–279; composition of, 231; control in, 230; and fear of failure, 241–242; and fear of losing control, 240–241; functioning of, 230–231; future issues of, 277–279; historical roles and responsibilities in, 234–237; leadership skills needed in, 239–240, 278; models of, 229–230; in new health care environment, 238–239; for organized delivery sys-

tems, 227–233; physician involvement in, 96–97, 109–110, 117–118, 120, 233, 256; selection of, dimensions of, 230–231; sensitivity of, to system, 228–229; streamlining, 242–243; structure of, 230; in study organizations, described, 252–254, 259–260, 267–268, 272–274; success factors in, 242–251; tradeoffs in, 279. *See also* Boards; Management structures; Physician leadership
Gretzsky, W., 34, 238
Griffith, J. R., 190, 227, 228, 233, 242
Group practice. *See* Physician groups

H

Hall, G., 189
Hambrick, D. C., 115
Hamel, G., 45
Hammer, M., 188
Handy, C., 29, 117
Hart, G. W., 309
Health assurance organization, 303, 304
Health care complexity, 46–47
Health care reform: approaches to, 3–5; community-building approach to, 5–8, 316; and ideal health system, 10–18. *See also* Change; Public policy
Health care system: costs of, 2; dominant logic in, 22–23; fragmentation of, 1–2; ideal, from health care executive's perspective, 14–17; ideal, key elements of, 17–18; ideal, from patient's perspective, 10–13; ideal, staging of, 30–35. *See also* Community health care management system; Health care reform
"Health Environmental Scan," 303, 305
Health maintenance, 22–23, 24–25; and physician-system integration, 147. *See also* Prevention-oriented care

Permission Credit Lines

Mr. Morris's story in "Scenario I" in Chapter Two comes from K. Lumsdon, "Crash Course, Piecing Together the Continuum of Care," *Hospitals & Health Networks*, November 20, 1994, pp. 26–28. Used with the permission of the publisher.

Mr. Dwight Taylor's story in "Scenario II" in Chapter Two comes from *Henry Ford Health System 1994 System Report*, written and published by Henry Ford Health System, 1994, Detroit, Mich., pp. 6, 8. Used with the permission of the publisher.

"The Daydream" and "The Harsh Reality" in Chapter Two comes from *Integration: Market Forces and Critical Success Factors*, published by Voluntary Hospitals of America, 1994, Irving, Texas, pp. 1–6. Used with the permission of the publisher.

The epigraph at the beginning of Chapter Four comes from F. Cerne, "Engineering a System Culture: Functioning as a System Cultivates Integration," *Hospitals & Health Networks*, 1994, 68(6), 36–39. Used with the permission of the publisher.

Fairview's mission statement in Chapter Five is used with the permission of Fairview Hospital and Healthcare Services.

The quote from J. L. Reinertsen in Chapter Six comes from "Living Guidelines," *Healthcare Forum Journal*, Nov./Dec. 1994, pp. 58–59. Used with the permission of the publisher.

The epigraph at the beginning of Chapter Seven comes from J. R. Griffith, "The Infrastructure of Integrated Delivery Systems," *Healthcare Executive*, May June 1995, pp. 12–17. Used with the permission of the publisher.

The "instrument panel" measure discussed in Chapter Seven comes from E. C. Nelson and others, "Report Cards or Instrument Panels: Who Needs What?" *Jt Comm J Qual Improv*, 1995, 21(4), 155–166. ©*Jt Comm J Qual Improv*. Oakbrook Terrace, Ill.: Joint Commission on Accreditation of Healthcare Organizations, 1995, 155–166. Reprinted with permission.